PERGAMON GENERAL PSYCHOLOGY SERIES

Editors: Arnold P. Goldstein, *Syracuse University*

Leonard Krasner, *SUNY, Stony Brook*

ADVANCES IN
EXPERIMENTAL CLINICAL PSYCHOLOGY

PGPS-17

ADVANCES
IN
EXPERIMENTAL
CLINICAL PSYCHOLOGY

Editors

Henry E. Adams

William K. Boardman

University of Georgia

PERGAMON PRESS

New York . Oxford . Toronto . Sydney . Braunschweig

Pergamon Press Inc., Maxwell House
Fairview Park, Elmsford, N. Y. 10523

Pergamon of Canada Ltd., 207 Queen's Quay West
Toronto 117, Ontario

Pergamon Press Ltd., Headington Hill Hall, Oxford

Pergamon Press (Aust.) Pty. Ltd., 19A Boundary Street
Rushcutters Bay, N. S. W.

Vieweg & Sohn GmbH., Burgplatz 1,
Braunschweig

Library of Congress Catalog No. 72-119600
Printed in the United States of America

08 016399 8

Educ.

Contents

Editors and Contributors

Henry E. Adams, *Ph.D.* is currently Professor of Psychology and Director of Clinical Training at The University of Georgia. His professional interests are in behavior therapy, psychophysiology, and neuropsychology. He is the author of numerous research and theoretical articles.

William K. Boardman, *Ph.D.* is Professor of Psychology and Director of The Psychology Clinic at The University of Georgia. His studies of perception and judgment as they relate to personality and psychopathology have appeared in several psychological journals.

Loren J. Chapman, *Ph.D.* is Professor of Psychology at The University of Wisconsin. His professional interests lie in the areas of cognitive functioning, psychodiagnosis, and psychosis.

Sidney E. Cleveland, *Ph.D.* is Chief, Psychology Service, Veterans Administration Hospital, Houston, Texas, and Clinical Professor of Psychology at Baylor College of Medicine and The University of Houston. He is co-author of the volume *Body Image and Personality* and author of numerous published scientific articles relating to body image, psychosomatic symptomatology, and life style.

Robert D. Hare, *Ph.D.* has been on the faculty at The University of British Columbia since 1963 and presently holds the rank of Associate Professor of Psychology. His research interests include psychophysiology, experimental research in personality, and the study of psychopathic behavior. His research on psychopathy won the Canadian Mental Health Association's 1969 research award of $25,000. Dr. Hare is the author of a book, *Psychopathy: Theory and Research.*

Brendan A. Maher, *Ph.D.* is currently Dean of the Graduate School at Brandeis University. His professional interests are in the areas of experimental psychopathology, conflict, autonomic responsiveness, and personality research. He is the author of numerous theoretical and research papers and has published several books, including *Principles of Psychopathology.*

Edward F. Zigler, *Ph.D.* is Director of the Child Development Training Program and a Professor in the Psychology Department, as well as Head of the Psychology Section in the Child Study Center of Yale University. He is a consultant to several governmental agencies and has served as a member of the National Planning and Steering Committee for Project Head Start. Professor Zigler was named the first Gunnar Dybwad Distinguished Scholar in the Behavioral and Social Sciences by the National Association for Retarded Children. He is the author of numerous theoretical and research papers.

Preface

The last 10 years have seen the development of a revolution in clinical psychology, a revolution which is not yet complete. The decade has been a period of scepticism and schisms. It has seen the widespread development of an attitude within the profession which was at first critical, and which progressed to a loss of faith in the traditional professional, theoretical, and technical procedures. Clinical psychologists have raised serious doubts about the validity of their assessment techniques, about the value of psychotherapy, and about the usefulness of clinical research which departs from accepted experimental methodology. One might say that once psychology lost its mind, and now clinical psychology has lost its faith.

This revolution has created many areas of uncertainty in the field of clinical psychology, and new schools of thought have arisen to fill them. These new points of view can be classified into three types of proposed solutions to the problems and the future of clinical psychology. The first position advocates the breaking of ties with academic research psychology, and the placing of emphasis on clinical orientation and on humanism. This view emphasizes that training in traditional academic and experimental psychology and its methods is irrelevant to the development and progress of clinical practice and training. Many psychologists who take this position feel that training in clinical psychology should no longer be conducted in universities, and have suggested the development of training centers in the form of independent professional schools. Such a move would handle the difficulties raised by the experimental evaluation of clinical procedures by divorcing clinical psychology from an experimental frame of reference, a tremendous price for the preservation of traditional clinical theory and methodology. The second position assumes an almost opposite point of view: that the uncertainties in theory and practice in clinical psychology are best resolved over time by increasing attention to the generation of useful clinical data through the application of traditional experimental methods. This opinion essentially favors tearing down clinical psychology's house of straw and rebuilding it in a manner more consistent with its academic and experimental foundation. The third position is more one of challenge than an attempt to solve clinical psychology's dilemma. It is a belief held by many of those clinical psychologists who feel that the profession cannot delay its response to society's needs at the community level. They take a position of action which breaks with traditional clinical methods, and which also runs ahead of experimental validation. They employ a flexible and pragmatic approach to social problems, while holding to the expectancy that future research will refine, stabilize, and validate the useful elements in their efforts.

The second and third positions have in common a commitment to the scientific method as a basic element of clinical psychology. The purpose of this book is to offer examples of how these latter approaches may yield information relevant to both professional and social problems.

The last 10 years have also been a period during which many exciting new developments in clinical psychology have begun to take shape. This series was designed to focus on the most promising of these research and theoretical developments in various areas of clinical psychology and to provide innovative psychologists with an opportunity to present their research projects and views without the limitations commonly imposed by scientific journals. It was decided by the editors that an individual, critical evaluation of each paper would not be given, in order to allow the reader to arrive at his own conclusions. Instead, a distinguished clinical psychologist was selected to evaluate briefly the materials presented by the contributors, to highlight new developments in the field, and to offer his views of the past, present, and probable future of clinical psychology. We were fortunate in having Brendan Maher assume this difficult task. He has given invaluable advice and aid throughout this project.

We would like to thank Joseph C. Hammock, former Head of the Department of Psychology; Robert A. McRorie, Assistant Vice President for Research and Director of General Research; H. Boyd McWhorter, Dean, College of Arts and Sciences; Mrs. Perrie Lou Bryant, Chief Secretary, Clinical Training Program; and other administrators and faculty at the University of Georgia whose cooperation and support have made this project possible. These papers were presented at the Georgia Symposium of Experimental Clinical Psychology at the University of Georgia in February 1969. This project was supported in part by the National Institute of Mental Health Training Grant No. *5 T01 MH 08924.*

Henry E. Adams and William K. Boardman
University of Georgia

Chapter 1

Psychopathic Behavior: Some Recent Theory and Research [1]

Robert D. Hare

Although history is replete with examples of behavior that we would now call psychopathic, it was not until the early nineteenth century that the concept of psychopathy began receiving some sort of formal recognition. In most cases, this recognition came from medical men who noticed that some disorders of behavior seemed to reflect a defect in moral rather than intellectual faculties. For example, in 1835 James Pritchard referred to a form of social and psychiatric abnormality in which:

> . . . the intellectual faculties appear to have sustained little or no injury, while the disorder is manifested principally or alone in the state of the feelings, temper, or habits. In cases of this description, the moral and active principles of the mind are strangely perverted and depraved; the power of self-government is lost or greatly impaired; and the individual is found to be incapable . . . of conducting himself with decency and propriety. (p. 4)

The disorders described by Pritchard were termed *moral insanity*, a concept that gave psychiatric recognition to the fact that an individual might be intellectually competent yet behaviorally abnormal. The concept was a broad one and included several types of neurosis, manic-depressive psychosis, neurotic forms of antisocial behavior, and behavior that we would now call psychopathic.

The transition from moral insanity to the concept of psychopathy as we know it was a stormy one, marked not only by confusion and argument concerning the nature of the disorders involved, but also by heated controversy about the usefulness of such concepts. Extended historical accounts of this transition have been given elsewhere (Craft, 1965; Dain & Carleson, 1962; Maughs, 1941; McCord & McCord, 1964; see also the bibliography by Hare & Hare, 1967) and need not be repeated here.

---

[1]Preparation of this manuscript was facilitated by Grant 609-7-163 from the National Health Grants Program (Canada) and by a research award from the Canadian Mental Health Association.

The Concept of Psychopathy

Although the term *psychopathy* has been used in a variety of contexts, there is a growing tendency among experimentally-oriented clinical psychologists to restrict its use to the clinical and behavioral syndrome so vividly described by Cleckley (1964) and Karpman (1961).

The main features of psychopathy, according to Cleckley, are as follows:

1. superficial charm and good intelligence,
2. absence of delusions and other signs of irrational thinking,
3. absence of nervousness or other neurotic manifestations,
4. unreliability,
5. untruthfulness and insincerity,
6. lack of remorse or shame,
7. antisocial behavior without apparent compunction,
8. poor judgment and failure to learn from experience,
9. pathologic egocentricity and incapacity for love,
10. general poverty in major affective reactions,
11. specific loss of insight,
12. unresponsiveness in general interpersonal relations,
13. fantastic and uninviting behavior with alcohol and sometimes without,
14. suicide rarely carried out,
15. sex life impersonal, trivial, and poorly integrated,
16. failure to follow any life plan.

Both Cleckley (1964) and Karpman (1961) describe the psychopath as a callous, emotionally immature, two-dimensional person who lacks the ability to experience the emotional components of personal and interpersonal behavior. He is able to *simulate* emotional reactions and affectional attachments when it will help him to obtain what he wants; however, he doesn't really *feel*. He experiences neither the psychological nor the physiological aspects of guilt and anxiety, although he may react with something like fear when his immediate comfort is threatened. His social and sexual relations with others are superficial, but demanding and manipulative. Future rewards and punishments do not exist, except in a very abstract and unreal way, with the result that they have little effect on his immediate behavior. His judgment is poor and often his behavior is guided entirely by impulse and current needs. His attempts to extricate himself from difficulty often result in an intricate and contradictory web of blatant lies, coupled with theatrical and sometimes convincing explanations and promises to change. Since the psychopath is egocentric, lacks empathy, and is unable to form warm emotional relationships with others, he tends to treat people as objects rather than as persons, and he experiences no guilt or remorse for having used them to satisfy his own needs.

The American Psychiatric Association (1952) term for the entity described by Cleckley and Karpman is *sociopathic personality disturbance, antisocial reaction,* defined as follows:

> This term refers to chronically antisocial individuals who are always in trouble, profiting neither from experience nor punishment, and maintaining no real loyalties to any person, group, or code. They are frequently callous and hedonistic, showing marked emotional immaturity, with lack of responsibility, lack of judgment, and an ability to rationalize their behavior so that it appears warranted, reasonable, and justified. (p. 38)

The term is cumbersome to use and, in practice, is often replaced by *sociopath.* The older and more familiar term *psychopath* still retains its popularity, however.[2]

When dealing with children, the Group for the Advancement of Psychiatry has proposed that the terms *tension-discharge disorder, impulse-ridden personality* be used in place of psychopathy or sociopathy, since the latter terms imply a personality pattern that is perhaps too fixed to apply to children. The impulse-ridden personality is described as follows:

> These children show shallow relationships with adults or other children, having very low frustration tolerance. They exhibit great difficulty in control of their impulses, both aggressive and sexual, which are discharged immediately and impulsively, without delay or inhibition, and often with little regard for the consequences. Little anxiety, internalized conflict, or guilt is experienced by most of these children, as the conflict remains largely external, between society and their impulses . . . The basic defect in impulse controls appears to be reinforced by a deficit in conscience or superego formation, with failure to develop the capacity for tension-storage and for the postponement of gratifications . . . Although their judgment and time concepts are poor, they usually have adequate intelligence and their reality testing in certain areas is quite effective. (Group for the Advancement of Psychiatry, 1966, pp. 247-48)

Secondary and Dysocial "Psychopathy"

The individual we have been discussing is sometimes referred to as the *primary, idiopathic,* or *classical* psychopath. These particular adjectives simply acknowledge the fact that many antisocial and aggressive acts are performed by individuals who are basically neurotic rather than psychopathic. Since the behavior of these individuals is assumed to be merely symptomatic of some emotional disturbance, they are sometimes called *secondary, symptomatic,* or *neurotic psychopaths.*

One of the difficulties with the use of terms like secondary and neurotic psychopathy is the implication that individuals so labeled are basically psychopaths. This is apt to be misleading, in my opinion, since the

---

[2]The 1968 revision of the APA's *Diagnostic and Statistical Manual of Mental Disorders* uses the term *antisocial personality.*

motivations behind their behavior, as well as their personality structure, life history, response to treatment, and prognosis, are probably quite different from those of the psychopath. Moreover, unlike psychopaths, these individuals are able to experience guilt and remorse for their behavior and to form meaningful, affectional relationships with others. Since their antisocial behavior is apparently motivated by neurotic conflicts and tensions, it may be more appropriate (at least until more data are available) to use terms that emphasize this neurotic element, e.g., *acting-out neurotic, neurotic delinquent*, etc. When dealing with children, the Group for Advancement of Psychiatry suggests that the term *neurotic personality disorder* be used.

Many individuals exhibit aggressive, antisocial behavior, not because they are psychopathic or emotionally disturbed, but because they have grown up in a delinquent subculture or in an environment that fosters and rewards such behavior. Their behavior, while considered deviant by society's standards, is nevertheless consonant with that of their own group, gang, or subculture. Although they are sometimes called *dysocial psychopaths*, they are unlike the "true" psychopath in that they are capable of strong loyalties, guilt, remorse, and warm relationships within the context of their own group. It therefore seems more appropriate to refer to them as *subcultural delinquents*. Where children are involved, the Group for the Advancement of Psychiatry prefers the term *sociosyntonic personality disorder*.

It is of considerable interest that the clinical subdivision of antisocial behavior into psychopathic, neurotic, and subcultural components is supported by several statistical studies of case history data. Jenkins, (1964, 1966), and his associates have repeatedly isolated several clusters of personality traits (or syndromes) occurring in delinquent children and in guidance clinic referrals. The three most common clusters have been labeled the *unsocialized-aggressive syndrome* (assaultive tendencies, starting fights, cruelty, defiance of authority, malicious mischief, inadequate guilt feelings); the *over-anxious syndrome* (seclusiveness, shyness, apathy, worrying, sensitiveness, submissiveness); and the *socialized delinquency syndrome* (bad companions, gang activities, cooperative stealing, habitual truancy from school and home, out late at night).

Other studies have produced similar results. Thus a series of factor analytic studies using behavior ratings (Quay, 1964b), case history data (Quay, 1964a), and responses to questionnaires (Peterson, Quay & Tiffany, 1961) has consistently yielded at least two main factors related to delinquency. The first factor, labeled *psychopathic delinquency*, reflects tough, amoral, and rebellious qualities coupled with impulsivity, distrust of authority, and freedom from family ties. The second factor, labeled *neurotic delinquency*, also reflects impulsive and aggressive tendencies; however, in this case, they are associated with tension, guilt, remorse, depression, and discouragement. A third factor has been identified in studies of personality questionnaires (Peterson *et al.*, 1961). Labeled *subcultural delinquency*, the factor reflects the attitudes and values commonly believed to occur in delinquent groups; it is similar to Jenkin's socialized delinquency syndrome and to the dysocial "psychopath" described above.

The results of several studies by Finney (e.g., 1966) provide further support for the distinction between psychopathic and neurotic forms of antisocial behavior. Using responses to a personality inventory, the MMPI, Finney isolated several factors, including one related to antisocial behavior and another related to anxiety, distress, and guilt. On the basis of his findings, Finney was able to distinguish between psychopathy (high in antisocial behavior, low in guilt), neurotic inhibition (low in antisocial behavior, high in guilt), and normalcy (low in antisocial behavior, low in guilt).

Although there is reasonably good agreement on the conceptual meaning of the term "psychopathy" (Albert, Brigante & Chase, 1959; Gray & Hutchison, 1964), it is, of course, not always so easy to identify those individuals who warrant the label "psychopathic". In this respect, the concept shares a problem that is common to all diagnostic categories, viz., the problem of diagnostic reliability (Phillips, 1968; Zubin, 1967). Nevertheless, as has been pointed out elsewhere (Hare, 1970), the problem is not as great as some would have us believe — certainly it is not great enough to prevent worthwhile research from being carried out. Moreover, the use of reasonably explicit criteria, such as those outlined by Cleckley, would seem to provide a useful starting point for the development of a more objective, empirically-based conceptualization of psychopathy.

Before reviewing some of the recent research and theory on psychopathy, there are several comments I'd like to make. First, compared to other disorders, e.g., schizophrenia, very little research on psychopathy has been carried out. This is unfortunate, but perhaps not too surprising. Most research is carried out in clinics and mental hospitals where the majority of patients are schizophrenic. Relatively few psychopaths are found in these institutions, and those who are there are likely to be considered nuisances rather than worthwhile subjects for research. Penal institutions provide the major source of psychopathic subjects, which leads to another problem — psychopathic criminals probably represent only a small proportion of the total population of psychopaths (Robins, 1966), viz., those whose behavior was unsuccessful (in a legal sense). Whether these individuals differ in important ways from those psychopaths whose behavior is legal or quasi-legal (though unethical and unscrupulous) is not known, although the possibility must be kept in mind when drawing conclusions from research that has used incarcerated psychopaths.

A second point is that there is as yet no well-developed, comprehensive theory of psychopathy. Instead, we have a large and diverse number of mini-theories and hypotheses, all of them incomplete or restricted to some selected aspect of psychopathy, and some of them untestable and without empirical foundation. At the same time, however, the elements of a general theory of psychopathy are beginning to emerge, largely as the result of the increasing use of procedures and conceptualizations derived from experimental psychology, including learning theory, motivation, and psychophysiology.

Finally, throughout the presentation to follow, I have avoided commenting upon the controversy over the most appropriate way of conceptualizing psychopathy. One viewpoint is that psychopathy is a relatively distinct clinical behavioral entity — a specific combination or clustering of characteristics that, individually and in other combinations, may be found in other disorders as well as in normal persons.

Many investigators, however, find it more appealing to conceptualize psychopathy in dimensional terms. According to this view, psychopaths as such do not exist, although some individuals may be considered more psychopathic than others if they occupy a more extreme position on some dimension that we choose to label "psychopathy". The difficulty here is that before we really can say that one person is more or less psychopathic than another, we need to know more of what the dimension consists. This means that we have to determine not only the psychological and physiological characteristics that define the dimension, but also their relative importance (the weights assigned them). An individual's position on the dimension would then be determined by the number of relevant characteristics he exhibits, their severity, and the weights assigned them. It should be possible, of course, to use multivariate statistical techniques to obtain information of this sort, and to derive a score or set of scores indicative of an individual's degree and type of psychopathy. To a certain extent, of course, the typologist already makes use of this procedure, but instead of identifying and weighing relevant characteristics empirically, he does so subjectively and on the basis of his experience.

Perhaps the disagreement about whether psychopathy is best viewed as a typology or as a dimensional concept arises because both views are appropriate, representing, as it were, the two sides of the same coin. It is also possible, as Zubin (1967) has put it, that, "The conflict between typology and dimensionality is a pseudoconflict dependent upon the state of knowledge of the field." (p. 398)

Research and Theory

Cortical Correlates of Psychopathy

The majority of the physiologically oriented studies of psychopathy have involved the electroencephalogram (EEG). In spite of their many limitations (e.g., inadequate control, ambiguous diagnosis of subjects, etc.), these studies have produced results that are too consistent to be ignored. The majority of studies have found that anywhere from 30 to 60% of diagnosed psychopaths exhibit some form of EEG abnormality, generally the presence of widespread slow-wave (4-7cps) activity. Since similar slow-wave activity is usually found in children, some investigators have suggested that psychopathy is associated with delayed cortical maturation (*see* Kiloh & Osselton, 1966). This *maturational retardation hypothesis* is quite appealing in its simplicity, and has some very indirect empirical support. For one thing, histologic studies of the nervous system at different ages does, in fact, suggest that cortical maturation is at least grossly correlated with the gradual shift from the slow-wave activity of childhood to the faster (alpha and beta) rhythms of adulthood (Lindsley, 1964; Scheibel & Scheibel, 1954). For another, there is evidence (Robins, 1966) that some psychopaths become less grossly antisocial with age, and that this improvement in behavior occurs most frequently between the ages of 30 and 40. It is possible, therefore, that the "burned-out" psychopath some clinicians talk about is the result of the delayed, but coincident, attainment of cortical and social maturation.

There are, of course, difficulties with this hypothesis. Although it is true that psychopaths and children have some characteristics in common — egocentricity, impulsivity, inability to delay gratification, etc. — the physiological and psychological processes involved are not necessarily the same. Moreover, the maturational retardation hypothesis does not take into account the tremendous effect that environmental experiences are likely to have upon the development and maintenance of psychopathy. And it does not explain why between 10 and 15% of the normal population also exhibit abnormal slow-waves and yet are mentally and behaviorally normal. It is possible, of course, that cortical immaturity *plus* some other organic and/or environmental factors are required to produce psychopathy.

Other interpretations of this slow-wave activity are possible. Several investigators have suggested that the normal alpha rhythm (around 10 cps) reflects cyclic fluctuations in the excitability or threshold for firing of cortical neurons (*see* review by Harter, 1967). They have also proposed that this excitability cycle may serve as a coding and gating mechanism for sensory input — only those impulses that arrive when a neuron or an aggregate of neurons is in an excitable state are able to fire the neurons and, therefore, to pass. The frequency of the excitability cycle may determine the upper limit at which incoming neural impulses can be transmitted. That is, neurons that reach their peak of excitability 10 times per second would permit more incoming impulses to pass (per minute of time) than would neurons that have a lower frequency cycle. What I am suggesting here is that it may be a low frequency excitability cycle that is represented by the slow-wave activity found in the EEGs of psychopaths. As a consequence of this low frequency cycle, there would be a tendency for the gating and attenuation of sensory input to be somewhat greater in psychopaths than in normal subjects. The results of a study by Shagass and Schwartz (1962) lead to much the same conclusion. These investigators used evoked potentials to determine the rate at which cortical neurons recovered from the effects of being fired. They found that psychopaths and schizophrenics exhibited slower cortical recovery than did neurotics and normals, a finding that is consistent with my suggestion that psychopaths may be characterized by a low frequency excitability cycle and a tendency to attenuate sensory input. Concerning the latter point, Shagass and Schwartz note that:

> Degree of recovery, as measured, appears to reflect the capacity of a neuronal aggregate to respond to stimuli following the first in a sequence. Impairment of the capacity to respond to later stimuli could result in failure to perceive the full range of cues available in a situation. (p. 50)

Slow neural recovery may also reflect a reduced state of cortical excitability (Pribram, 1967) and, by implication, cortical underarousal. I'll come back to this point later.

There is some evidence that extremely impulsive and aggressive psychopaths exhibit EEG abnormalities that are more specific and localized than the diffuse slow-wave activity already mentioned. Hill (1952) found, for example, that about 14% of 194 severely aggressive psychopaths exhibited abnormal slow-wave activity in the temporal lobes of the cerebral hemispheres. The incidence of this activity was considerably lower in normal subjects (2% of 146), schizophrenics (4.8% of 147), inmates of a prison (2.8% of 143), and murderers (8.2% of 110). Within the psychopathic group, there was a strong tendency for the incidence of this temporal abnormality to be much greater in the highly aggressive than in the less aggressive subjects. More recently, Bay-Rakal (1965) found that temporal slow-wave activity in behavior problem children was related to developmental delay, poor control of impulses, and inadequate socialization.

There is some evidence that another form of temporal lobe abnormality, *positive spikes*, also may be related to impulsive and aggressive forms of psychopathy. Positive spikes are bursts of 6-8 cps and 14-16 cps activity apparently emanating from the limbic system and the temporal areas of the brain (Hughes, 1965). While the incidence of positive spikes in the general population is very low (1-2%), it may be as high as 30 or 40% in explosively impulsive and aggressive individuals, including psychopaths (Kurland, Yeager & Arthur, 1963). The behavior of patients with positive-spike activity can be very dramatic indeed (*see* Schwade & Geiger, 1965). Typically, the patient has a history of impulsive behavior and "overwhelming" aggressive urges. The behavioral act or "attack" is often precipitated by relatively trivial, innocuous situations, and once started cannot be stopped until its completion. In spite of its destructiveness, positive-spike behavior is generally coordinated and well-directed and is often performed with considerable skill and precision.

Most investigators have observed that, at the completion of the act, the individual expresses no guilt, anxiety, or remorse for what he has done, although he is often able to discuss it on a verbal level.

Now I'm not too certain about how important these localized EEG abnormalities are in helping us understand psychopathy. For one thing, the observation of an abnormality in an EEG recording does not necessarily mean there is a corresponding brain abnormality; nor, for that matter, does a normal EEG always indicate the absence of brain disorder (Kiloh & Osselton, 1964). Further, many other individuals, and not all psychopaths, exhibit these localized abnormalities. Nevertheless, I think we should at least consider the possibility that these abnormalities in the more highly impulsive and aggressive forms of psychopathy reflect some sort of dysfunction in underlying temporal and limbic mechanisms. Consider, for example, the following line of reasoning which, though highly speculative, is consistent with the EEG findings already discussed, and also with recent research on experimentally induced brain lesions.

Although the limbic system and associated mechanisms are complex and their functions not yet well-understood, it is known that they are involved in sensory and memory processes and in the central regulation of emotional and motivational behavior. For our purposes, it is sufficient to note that the limbic system appears to have both facilitatory and inhibitory effects upon behavior; that is, activity in some mechanisms facilitates and maintains ongoing behavior; activity in other mechanisms inhibits or disrupts ongoing behavior (see Grossman, 1967; McCleary, 1966). These limbic mechanisms appear to play a particularly important role in the regulation of fear-motivated behavior, including learning to inhibit a response in order to avoid punishment (passive-avoidance learning). Research reviewed by McCleary (1966), for instance, indicates that lesions in the limbic inhibitory mechanisms make it difficult to learn to inhibit a punished response. A more general effect of these lesions may be to produce perseveration of the most dominant response in a given situation. That is, the response with the greatest tendency to occur (either because of some inherent tendency or because of past learning experiences) will occur, even though it had previously been inhibited because of punishment.

On the basis of this research, we might hypothesize that the temporal slow-wave activity, frequently observed in the EEG records of highly impulsive psychopaths, reflects a malfunction of some limbic inhibitory mechanism and that this malfunction makes it difficult to learn to inhibit behavior that is likely to lead to punishment.[3] This malfunction could be due

---

[3] Douglas (1967), in a recent review, suggests that slow-wave activity is associated with a reduction in the inhibitory function of one of the limbic areas, the hippocampus.

to hereditary or experiential factors or, more likely, to injury, disease, or to biochemical or vascular changes which temporarily dampen the inhibiting activity of important mechanisms. According to McCleary's concept of response perseveration, the result would be that the most dominant response in any given situation would tend to occur regardless of its consequences. For example, the tendency to engage in some form of sexual behavior generally increases when sexual drives are high (because of prolonged sexual deprivation, the presence of sex-related cues, etc.). The actual form that sexual behavior takes depends upon such things as learning, the nature of the opportunities available, and so on. But even though response tendencies of a sexual kind are dominant, they may, in fact, be inhibited because of social restrictions, unwillingness of the intended partner, fear of pregnancy, disease, or sexual inadequacy. If we assume that the effectiveness of such inhibitions is dependent upon the normal functioning of limbic inhibitory mechanisms, and if we further assume that under certain conditions (e.g., under high drive states) these mechanisms malfunction in the psychopath, we would then predict that, given the urge, he would initiate and complete the act. The clinical comments that the psychopath's behavior is impulsive and determined more by his immediate needs than by possible consequences could thus be interpreted in terms of the failure of the appropriate inhibitory mechanisms to function properly.

Autonomic Correlates of Psychopathy

Many of the psychopath's characteristics — his apparent lack of anxiety, guilt, or remorse, his inability to empathize with others, his shallow emotional involvements, his failure to be influenced by threatened punishment, etc. — presumably have emotional and hence, autonomic correlates. It is not surprising, therefore, that many investigators have attempted to relate psychopathy to some form of disturbance or anomaly in the functioning of the autonomic nervous system. Since these attempts have been reviewed elsewhere (Hare, 1968a, 1970), only a brief summary, along with some more recent research, will be given here.

Several investigators have obtained measures of autonomic activity from subjects that were in a resting state, i.e., in a state of relative quiescence. Their findings are summarized in Table I. It is apparent that all of the significant differences between groups, as well as most of the trends toward a difference, were confined to two aspects of electrodermal activity — palmar skin conductance (SC) and spontaneous or non-specific fluctuations in skin conductance (NSP). And most of these studies used relatively well-defined groups of psychopaths (designated as Group P in Table I).

The results of these studies indicate that psychopaths may have a lower level of resting skin conductance than do nonpsychopaths. Psychopaths also appear to be characterized by a relatively low level of spontaneous

Table I

Resting Tonic Level in Psychopaths

Investigator	Subjects [a]	Variables [b]	Findings
Lindner (1942)	M, NPC	SR, HR, RR	No significant difference.
Ruilmann & Gulo (1950)	M, NC	SR, HR, RR, BP	No significant difference.
Lykken (1955)	P, M, NC	SR	Group P had lowest SR.
Fox & Lippert (1963)	M, NPC	SC, NSP	Group M gave fewer NSP.
Schachter & Latané (1964)	P, NPC	HR	No significant difference.
Goldstein (1965)	M, NC	SC, HR, RR, BP, MAPs	No significant difference.
Hare (1965b)	P, NPC, NC	SC	Group P had lowest SC.
Hare (1965c)	P, NPC	SC	Group P had lower SC.
Lippert & Senter (1966)	M, NPC	SC, NSP	No significant difference, though trend towards fewer NSP in Group M.
Hare (1968a)	P, M, NPC	SC, NSP, HR, P-T, RR	Groups P and M had lower SC than Group NPC; tendency for Group P to be lowest on NSP and P-T.

[a] P=Psychopaths; M=mixed group of subjects; NPC=nonpsychopathic criminals or patients; NC=noninstitutionalized subjects.
[b] SR=skin resistance; SC=skin conductance; NSP=nonspecific or spontaneous GSRs; HR=heart rate; RR=respiration rate; BP=blood pressure; P-T=peak-trough difference in HR; MAPs=muscle action potentials; NVC=nonspecific or spontaneous peripheral vasoconstriction; VC=peripheral vasoconstriction.

Table I (Continued)

Resting Tonic Level in Psychopaths

Investigator	Subjects [a]	Variables [b]	Findings
Schalling, Lidberg, Levander & Dahlin, (1968)	P, NPC, SC	SC, NSP, NVC	Group P had lower NSP and tendency toward lower SC.

[a] P=Psychopaths; M=mixed group of subjects; NPC=nonpsychopathic criminals or patients; NC=noninstitutionalized subjects.

[b] SR=skin resistance; SC=skin conductance; NSP=nonspecific or spontaneous GSRs; HR=heart rate; RR=respiration rate; BP=blood pressure; P-T=peak-trough difference in HR; MAPs=muscle action potentials; NVC=nonspecific or spontaneous peripheral vasoconstriction; VC=peripheral vasoconstriction.

electrodermal activity — the differences between groups were not always significant, but the trends were consistent.[4] Since both measures of electrodermal activity may reflect the level of sympathetic arousal, these findings provide some support for the hypothesis that psychopaths are sympathetically underaroused while in a relative state of rest. Figure 1 gives some idea of the changes in electrodermal activity (and hence, arousal) that can occur throughout the course of an experiment. Skin conductance and spontaneous electrodermal responses were measured after a 15-minute resting period and after hearing a series of repetitive, moderately intense tones for 15 minutes. It is obvious that, throughout the course of the experiment, the psychopaths became even less aroused while the nonpsychopaths became more aroused.

The situation with respect to autonomic responsivity is somewhat more complex (Table II). In general, psychopaths give normal electrodermal responses (GSRs) to simple stimuli such as lights and tones, but they are relatively unresponsive to stimuli preceding shock, i.e., to the threat of shock.

---

[4] It is possible that psychopaths exhibit less *autonomic* variability generally than do nonpsychopaths. In one of my studies (Hare, 1968a), spontaneous fluctuations in electrodermal activity (NSP) and in heart rate (P-T) were combined in a multivariate analysis to provide a composite measure of autonomic variability. The results indicated that autonomic variability in psychopaths was significantly less than it was in nonpsychopaths, even though the difference between groups in the components of autonomic variability (NSP and P-T) were, by themselves, not significant.

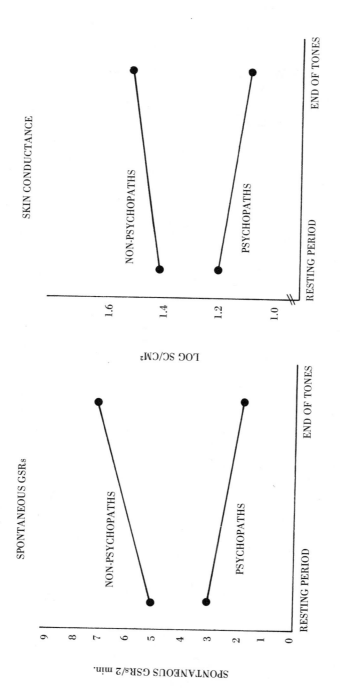

Figure 1

Electrodermal activity near the beginning (resting period) of the experiment and after a series of repetitive tones. Based upon Hare (1968a).

Table II

Autonomic Responsivity in Psychopaths

Investigator	Subjects[a]	Variables[b]	Stimuli	Findings
Lindner (1942)	M, NPC	SC, HR, RR	Tones & shock	No significant difference.
Ruilmann & Gulo (1950)	N, NC	SC, HR, RR, BP	"Sensory stimuli", questions, arithmetic problems	Group M showed less GSR responsivity.
Lykken (1955)	P, M, NC	SR	Tones & shock; lie detection	Groups P and M showed less GSR responsivity to shock, tones signaling shock, and "lying".
Gellhorn (1957)	M, NPC	BP	Injection of mecholyl	Group M showed smaller BP drop and quicker homeostatic recovery.
Tong (1959)	M, NC	SR	Heat, tones, tactile, frustration	Some group M more responsive, some less.
Schachter & Latané (1964)	P, NPC	HR	Injection of adrenalin	Group P more responsive.
Goldstein (1965)	M, NC	SC, HR, RR, BP, Maps	White noise	No significant difference.
Hare (1965b)	P, NPC, NC	SC	Shock and threat of shock	No significant difference in responsivity to shock; Group P least responsive to threat of shock.
Hare (1965c)	P, NPC	SC	Tones & shock	No significant difference in responsivity to shock; Group P less responsive to tones signaling shock.
Lippert & Senter (1966)	M, NPC	SC, NSP	Lights, tones, threatened shock.	No significant difference to light & tones; Group M less responsive to threat of shock.

Table II (Cont)

Autonomic Responsivity in Psychopaths

Investigator	Subjects[a]	Variables[b]	Stimuli	Findings
Hare (1968a)	P, M, NPC	SC, HR, VC	Tones	No significant difference in GSR responsivity; Group P showed smallest cardiac deceleration to novel tones, and slower habituation of cardiac and vasomotor responses.
Schalling, Lidberg, Levander & Dahlin (1968)	P, NP	SC, NSP, NVC	Tones	Group P gave fewer NSP.

[a,b] Same as for Table I.

Several studies have also found that they give normal GSRs to electric shock, although it is difficult to draw any firm conclusions here because, in each case, the shock was preceded by a warning signal, i.e., some sort of classical conditioning paradigm was involved. Kimmel (1966) has reviewed evidence suggesting that when a conditioned stimulus (CS) is followed by an unconditioned stimulus (UCS) such as shock, the CS eventually exerts an inhibitory influence on the unconditioned response (UCR) elicited by the shock. That is, the response to a shock preceded by a signal is smaller than it would have been had the shock been presented alone. This means that in those studies in Table II which used a signal-shock combination, electro-dermal responsivity to shock was probably confounded with the inhibitory influence of the signal. It is conceivable that this inhibitory influence is either greater (or less) than that shown by nonpsychopaths. Obviously, more research is needed in which noxious stimuli are presented both with and without a warning signal.

A recent study (Hare, 1968a) was concerned with the psychopath's autonomic responsivity and rate of habituation to simple stimulation. This is the same study already referred to in Figure 1. After the 15-minute resting period, subjects heard a series of 15 identical tones. They were then presented with a 16th tone, lower in frequency and intensity than the preceding 15 tones. The mean electrodermal response shown by each group to the 15 repetitive tones and to the novel 16th tone is plotted in Figure 2.

It is apparent that there were no appreciable differences between groups, either in the magnitude of GSR elicited by the tones or in the rate at which GSR magnitude decreased (habituated) with repeated stimulation. By way of contrast, consider what happened when cardiovascular changes were assessed. (The heart rate response to stimulation that is not too intense or noxious is generally one of deceleration.) The mean deceleration in heart rate shown by each group to the 16 tones is plotted in Figure 3. Two things are of interest here: the first being the relatively small response given by the psychopaths (Group P) to tones that could be considered novel or unfamiliar (Tones 1 and 16). The second point is that the response habituated more slowly for the psychopaths than for the nonpsychopaths (Group NP).

Data were also available on a second cardiovascular variable, peripheral (finger) vasoconstriction. The results are shown in Figure 4. While the differences between groups were small and the responses quite variable, the psychopaths tended to give the largest responses, particularly during Tones 13-15.[5]

These results may not be as confusing as they appear at first glance. Several interpretations are possible, including one that is based upon the Russian conception of the *orienting response*, (Lynn, 1966; Sokolov, 1963). The orienting response (OR) is a nonspecific, complex response to changes in stimulation. It includes turning the sensory receptors toward the source of the stimulation, blocking of the EEG alpha rhythm, peripheral vasoconstriction, cephalic vasodilation, increase in skin conductance (GSR), pupil dilation, cardiac deceleration, and an increase in muscle tension. One effect of the OR is apparently to increase sensitivity to novel or unfamiliar stimulation. If the stimulus is repetitive and without special significance to the organism, the OR habituates, but returns when a novel stimulus is presented.

It is obvious from inspection of Figures 2-4 that all groups gave the appropriate GSR components of the OR, but that psychopaths gave comparatively small cardiac ORs, especially to the novel 16th tone. A tentative conclusion, based upon the cardiac data, might be that psychopaths

---

[5]I recently reanalyzed some of the data in this study. Six variables (resting skin conductance, resting non-specific GSRs, resting fluctuations in heart rate, cardiac deceleration to Tone 16, cardiac habituation rate, and the difference between cardiac deceleration to Tones 15 and 16) were combined in a multiple discriminant analysis. The combined difference between psychopaths (Group P) and non-psychopaths (Group NP) was highly significant, F (6/25) = 23.57, $p < .001$. Of the 32 Ss involved in the analysis, 26 were correctly classified.

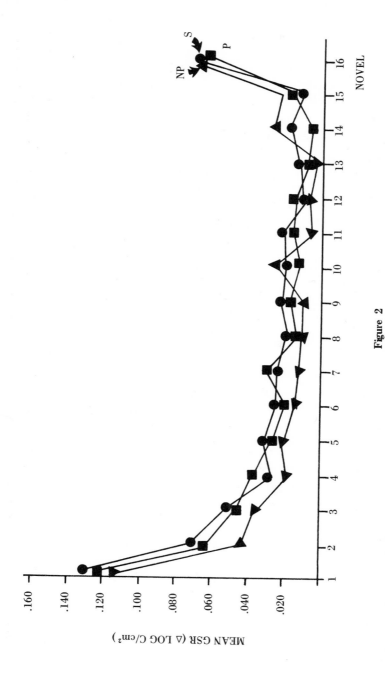

Figure 2

Mean GSR to repetitive (Tones 1-15) and novel (Tone 16) stimulation. P = psychopaths; S = mixed group; NP = nonpsychopaths. From Hare (1968a), *J. Abnorm. Psychol.*, 73, No. 3. Reprinted with permission of American Psychological Association.

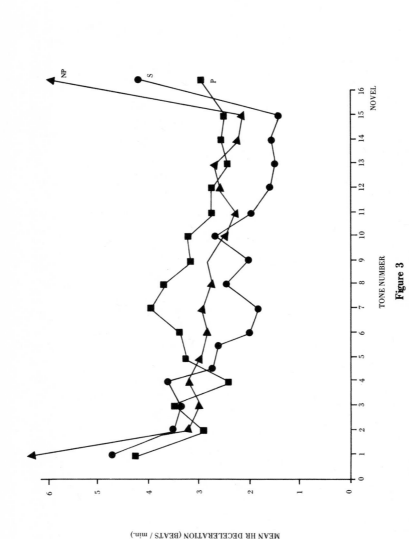

Figure 3

Mean cardiac deceleration to repetitive (Tones 1-15) and novel (Tone 16) stimulation. P = psychopaths; S = mixed group; NP = nonpsychopaths. From Hare (1968a), *J. Abnorm. Psychol.*, 73, No. 3. Reprinted with permission of American Psychological Association.

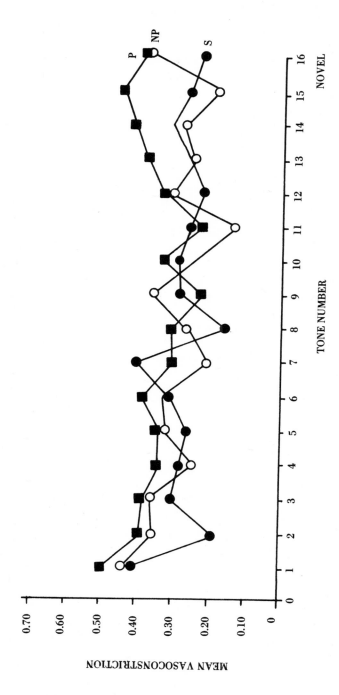

Figure 4

Mean peripheral vasoconstriction to repetitive (Tones 1-15) and novel (Tone 16) stimulation. P = psychopaths; S = mixed group; NP = nonpsychopaths. From Hare (1968a),*J. Abnorm. Psychol.*,73, No. 3. Reprinted with permission of American Psychological Association.

are less attentive and sensitive to small changes in environmental stimulation than is the more normal person. Recall that the cortical studies discussed earlier led to the same conclusion.

A second (and related) interpretation of these findings is suggested by the results of a study by McDonald, Johnson, and Hord (1964). These investigators also observed the rate at which various components of the OR habituated. They found that when their subjects were divided, on the basis of EEG criteria, into those who showed signs of drowsiness during the experiment and those who did not, different habituation patterns emerged. Briefly, the GSR, cardiac, and vasoconstrictive responses of their drowsy and alert subjects were remarkably similar, respectively, to those of the psychopaths and nonpsychopaths in my study. What this suggests is that these psychopaths may have become progressively more drowsy and less cortically and autonomically aroused than did the other subjects. That psychopaths do, in fact, tend to become drowsy during tedious experiments has been suggested by several investigators. Forssman and Frey (1953), for example, found that psychopathic boys not only exhibited a high incidence of slow-wave activity in their EEGs, but also tended to fall asleep more readily during the examination than did other boys. On the basis of these findings, Forssman and Frey suggested that psychopathy is characterized by a wavering or decrement in attentiveness. In commenting on this study, Stern and McDonald (1965) raised the additional possibility that the tendency of psychopaths to become drowsy in experimental situations may reflect the fact that these situations generate less stress or anxiety than is the case with normal subjects. The autonomic data reported earlier (Figure 1) are, of course, consistent with this suggestion.

Psychopathy, Arousal, and Need for Stimulation

Cleckley (1964) says of the psychopath:

> Being bored, he will seek to cut up more than the ordinary person in order to relieve the tedium of his unrewarding existence (p. 426) . . . Perhaps the emptiness or superficiality of a life without major goals or deep loyalties, or real love, would leave a person with high intelligence and other superior qualities so bored that he would eventually turn to hazardous, self-damaging, outlandish, antisocial, and even destructive exploits in order to find something fresh and stimulating in which to apply his useless and unchallenged energies and talents. (p.44)

Many other clinicians have similarly commented that the psychopath seems unable to tolerate routine and boredom and that he is constantly seeking new and exciting things to do. It is of some interest, therefore, that quite a few empirical studies not only lead to more or less the same conclusions, but, in addition, provide hypotheses about the *reasons* for these aspects of psychopathy (Hare, 1970). One hypothesis is that the psychopath is in a chronic state of cortical underarousal and that he attempts to increase arousal to some more optimal level by seeking stimulation with "exciting" qualities (Eysenck, 1967; Hare, 1968a; Quay, 1965). A related hypothesis is that sensory input is somehow attenuated, with the result that a greater amount of stimulation is required to attain this optimal level of arousal (Eysenck, 1967; Hare, 1968a; Petrie, 1967).

As used here, arousal is a dimension representing the physiological and psychological state of an organism. The low end of the dimension is characterized by deep sleep, complete loss of awareness, and a low level of physiological activity. As arousal increases, the individual's awareness of the environment and his behavioral efficiency also increase, but only up to a point — beyond some optimal level of arousal, awareness and efficiency tend to break down. The function relating arousal and behavioral efficiency, often described as an "inverted U function" (Malmo, 1966), is presented in Figure 5. States of arousal above and below some optimal level are related to progressive decreases in the efficiency of behavior. A similar relationship probably exists between arousal and affective experience — both high and low levels of arousal are more unpleasant than some more moderate level. One implication of this latter relationship is that an individual in a low state of arousal will likely seek to *increase* arousal, while one who is in a heightened state of arousal will likely seek to *decrease* it. Similarly, changes in arousal toward this optimal level (either from above or below) ought to be rewarding, while changes away from this level ought to be punishing. One of the most important determinants of arousal is, of course, stimulation (the sensory pathways send collaterals into the reticular formation which, in turn, sends diffuse excitatory impulses to the cortex), and we would, therefore, expect an individual to either seek stimulation or avoid it, depending upon whether he is below or above what is for him an optimal level of arousal for the particular situation in which he finds himself.

What I am suggesting here is that the environmental conditions that permit a normal person to enjoy an optimal level of arousal result in the psychopath being below an optimal level.[6] The evidence for this suggestion is

_____

[6] In many respects, Eysenck's (1967) theory of personality bears upon arousal conceptions of psychopathy. For example, one of the main personality dimensions in his theory is *extroversion*, a dimension that he has recently related to reticular-cortical arousal — extroverts fall at the low end and introverts at the high end of the arousal continuum. In terms of cortical arousal then, extroverts and psychopaths appear to be similar. Eysenck does, in fact, refer to the psychopath as a "neurotic extrovert." The difficulty here lies in his use of the adjective "neurotic". In Eysenck's theory, *neuroticism* or emotionality is related to lability of the autonomic nervous system. However, the evidence is contrary to his contention that psychopaths are autonomically labile. This discrepancy may reflect the fact that what Eysenck refers to as "psychopaths" are, in fact, neurotic delinquents — within the context of his theory, psychopaths in the Cleckley sense could more appropriately be referred to as "stable extroverts". At the same time, however, the analogy between extroversion and psychopathy shouldn't be pushed too far — psychopathy involves a great deal more than cortical underarousal. Moreover, several studies (e.g., Schoenherr, 1964) have found that psychopaths are neither extroverted nor neurotic in the Eysenckian sense.

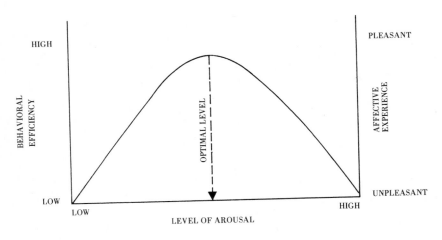

Figure 5

Hypothetical curve relating level of arousal to behavioral efficiency and affective experience.

mostly indirect but, nevertheless, quite consistent. Some of this evidence has already been presented. To recapitulate briefly, the psychopath's slow neural recovery from the effects of stimulation (Shagass & Schwartz, 1962), his "low frequency cortical excitability cycle", his tendency to become drowsy during experimental routine and to exhibit a pattern of autonomic responsivity similar to that found in drowsy subjects, all lead to the conclusion that, in the situations involved, he is in a relatively reduced state of cortical arousal. The finding (Rose, 1964) that psychopathic patients have a higher two-flash threshold than do more anxious patients leads to the same conclusion. Some of the previously discussed findings on autonomic activity also lead to this conclusion. Of particular interest here is the tendency for the psychopath to exhibit a relatively low degree of *autonomic variability* — that is, spontaneous fluctuations in skin conductance and heart rate. Lacey and Lacey (1958) have found that fluctuations in autonomic activity represent a reliable individual characteristic, and have postulated that there is an intimate coupling between these fluctuations and cortical activity. For example, although autonomic, cortical, and behavioral arousal may become dissociated under some conditions (Lacey, 1967), fluctuations in autonomic activity may have excitatory effects which, functioning via "hypothalamic-cortical discharge and possibly via visceral afferent feedback, would be expected to produce an increment in the level of cortical arousal, which would be self-sustaining for some time" (Lacey & Lacey, 1958, pp. 169-70). The tendency of psychopaths to exhibit relatively little autonomic variability during rest may, therefore, mean that in the absence of fairly salient stimulation, they are autonomically and cortically underaroused.

Now if psychopaths are, in fact, cortically underaroused, that is, below an optimal level of arousal, they should show a marked tendency to seek stimulation, thereby increasing arousal. This expectation is supported by the findings that they prefer "frightening" activities to those that are safe but dull (Lykken, 1955); that they have a preference for novel and complex stimulation (Skrzypek, 1969); that they perform better with large amounts of stimulation (Currie, 1965) and with stimulus onset rather than offset (Wiesen, 1965); and that they do poorly in a tedious vigilance task (Orris, 1967).

There are, of course, many other ways in which psychopaths could increase cortical arousal. One way would be to resort to all forms of self-generated stimulation, including fantasy and daydreams, when appropriate sources of external stimulation are not available. Incidentally, I think that, if we examine the content of their fantasies, we will find that psychopaths are concerned with "exciting" themes rather than with mental planning. This would help to account for some of their poor judgment and lack of foresight, assuming (cf. Singer, 1966) that one of the functions of fantasy is to permit "vicarious trial and error" in which various courses of action and their possible consequences are run through mentally beforehand.

Besides self-generated stimulation, psychopaths should show a marked preference for psychotomimetic drugs (such as LSD-25, mescaline, psilocybin) and drugs that are psychomotor stimulants (e.g. amphetamine, methadrine). They should also find the intense and varied visual, auditory, and kinesthetic stimulation associated with psychedelic music and dancing very appealing.

Earlier, I suggested that psychopathy might be characterized by a tendency for sensory input to be gated out or attenuated. If the psychopath's sensory input is, in fact, subject to a certain degree of attenuation during transmission, a given amount of stimulation would tend to move him a shorter distance up the arousal continuum than it would the normal person. The psychopath would thus not only need stimulation, but, when he receives it, he would find that it does not increase arousal very much (at least not as much as it would if he were a normal person). The result would be even more of a tendency to seek new and exciting stimulation than if he were simply cortically underaroused.

There could be other consequences of a general tendency to attenuate sensory input. For one thing, many of the cues essential to adequate social functioning are subtle and of low intensity. The psychopath's tendency to attenuate input would mean that some of these cues would be below threshold and ineffective. Furthermore, in an attempt to attain an optimal level of arousal, he would actively seek intense stimulation, or at least stimulation that has exciting or arousing properties. In scanning the environment for such stimulation, however, he would probably miss, or perhaps ignore, many social cues — cues that have important informational and emotional content and are necessary for the guidance of behavior. As a result, he would ordinarily be little influenced by many of the cues emanating, for example, from other individuals — signs of distress, personal hurt, approval, disapproval, etc. If, however, these cues had some special significance for him — as would be the case if he was trying to use others to satisfy his own needs — we might expect that the psychopath would make a special effort to attend to them more closely.

Another consequence of a tendency to attenuate sensory input is that psychopaths should be less sensitive to very weak stimulation but more tolerant of strong stimulation than are normal persons.[7] Hare (1968b) and Schoenherr (1964) did, in fact, find that psychopaths had higher shock detection thresholds than did nonpsychopaths; however, a study recently conducted by one of my students (Hare & Thorvaldson, 1970) failed to support these findings. A similar (equivocal) situation holds with respect to tolerance for intense stimulation. Schalling and Levander (1964) found that nonanxious psychopathic delinquents had higher pain and tolerance thresholds than did anxious, nonpsychopathic delinquents. Several other studies, however, have found no significant differences between psychopathic and nonpsychopathic criminals, either in tolerance for shock (Hare, 1965c, 1966a; Schoenherr, 1964) or in the ratings of the "painfulness" of shock of given intensity (Schachter & Latané, 1964). It is possible that these discrepant findings reflect subject and procedural differences, as well as the failure to take motivational variables into account. Obviously, the point at which an individual says "that's enough" represents not how much shock he *can* tolerate, but only how much he is *willing* to tolerate under the particular conditions of the situation in which he happens to find himself. Presumably, the use of appropriate incentives would increase the intensity of shock willingly tolerated. On the assumption that these incentives would have a greater effect on psychopaths than on nonpsychopaths, Hare and Thorvaldson (1970) determined tolerance levels under two conditions. In the first condition, subjects were simply asked to indicate when the shock was the strongest they could take. Following this, cigarettes were used to induce the subjects to accept more intense shock. The results are plotted in Figure 6. There were no significant differences between groups when incentives were not used; however, with cigarettes as an incentive, the psychopaths were willing to accept much more shock than were the nonpsychopaths.

---

[7] Similar predictions concerning extroverts have long been made by Eysenck (1967).

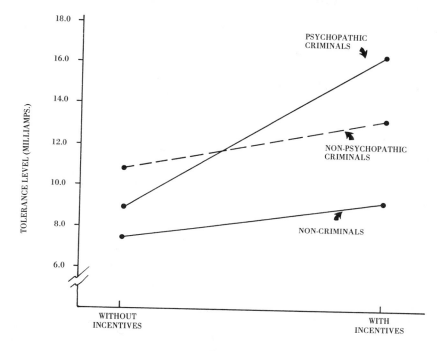

Figure 6

Intensity of shock tolerated with and without incentives. (N = 14 each group). From Hare & Thorvaldson (1970). *J. Abnorm. Psychol.* Reprinted with permission of American Psychological Association.

Psychopathy and Learning

Since an extensive review of the relationship between psychopathy and learning has been given elsewhere (Hare, 1970), only a brief summary of the main findings is needed here.

Intelligence tests. A considerable number of studies indicate that psychopaths are not deficient in the intellectual processes and the learning experiences that are reflected in standard tests of intelligence (e.g., Craddick, 1961; Gurvitz, 1950).

Rote verbal learning. Although several investigators have found that psychopaths perform poorly on a serial learning task (Fairweather, 1953) and that they exhibit less retroactive inhibition than do normal persons (Sherman, 1957), other investigators (Kadlub, 1956; Schoper, 1958) could not replicate these findings.

Verbal conditioning. Some investigators (e.g., Johns & Quay, 1962; Quay & Hunt, 1965) have reported that psychopathic criminals do not condition as readily as do neurotic criminals; however, their data were not very convincing. Other investigators have found that psychopaths condition as well (Blaylock, 1960; Bryan & Kapche, 1967) or better (Bernard & Eisenman, 1967) than do other subjects.

Probability learning. Painting (1961) found that psychopaths did well in a probability learning experiment when the correct response on any given trial was either randomly determined or was dependent upon the trial immediately preceding. However, they did poorly when the correct response was dependent upon what had happened *two* trials earlier, indicating, perhaps, that psychopaths have difficulty in perceiving the contingencies between past events and the consequences of their present behavior.

Thus far, the evidence for differences between psychopaths and normal persons is not very impressive. However, when classical conditioning and avoidance learning studies are considered, more consistent differences do become apparent. Because of their importance to several theories of psychopathy, these studies will be discussed in somewhat more detail.

Classical conditioning. The published research has been confined to eyeblink and electrodermal (GSR) conditioning. With respect to the former, and using a simple conditioning paradigm (only one CS), Miller (1966) found that psychopathic criminals were not significantly inferior to neurotic criminals and noncriminals in the acquisition of a conditioned eyeblink. Warren and Grant (1955), using college students with high and low scores on the *Psychopathic Deviate (Pd)* scale of the MMPI, obtained similar results. However, when a differential conditioning paradigm was used (one stimulus, the CS^+, was followed by the UCS, an airpuff; the other stimulus, the CS^-, was not), the low-*Pd* subjects showed differential conditioning, whereas the high-*Pd* subjects did not. The latter apparently failed to develop conditioned discrimination because of their tendency to avoid the discomfort associated with the airpuff by blinking indiscriminately to both the CS^+ and the CS^-. The implication here seems to be that the responses of some of the high-*Pd* subjects were partially voluntary in nature.

The results with electrodermal conditioning, using electric shock as the unconditioned stimulus (UCS), have been more consistent. Lykken (1955) found that psychopaths exhibit poor differential GSR conditioning; similar results have been obtained with a simple conditioning paradigm (Hare, 1965b), as well as with a form of long-delay conditioning (Hare, 1965c, 1965d). Since these studies involved strong electric shock as the UCS and a sympathetic response (GSR) as the CR, the results have generally been taken as support for the hypothesis that psychopaths are defective at fear conditioning. As we'll see shortly, this hypothesis is an important one in accounting for their failure to avoid punishment. In the meantime, it is worth noting that these conditioning studies of psychopathy are somewhat limited in scope since they involved only noxious stimuli (shock) and only one dependent variable (GSR). The result is that they tell us nothing, except by inference, about whether psychopaths condition poorly when other classes of UCS and other autonomic variables are involved. Preliminary results from a study by one of my doctoral students, Michael Quinn, partially overcome these limitations. Quinn used a delayed, differential paradigm in which three noticeably different conditioned stimuli (tones) were presented 16 times each, in random order. Each tone was 10 seconds long; the termination of two of the tones was accompanied by either a strong electric shock $(CS^+ \text{-}S)$ or a two-second slide of a nude female $(CS^+ \text{-}P)$; no UCS followed the third tone (C^-). The subjects included 18 psychopathic criminals (Group P), carefully selected on the basis of Cleckley's criteria, and 18 nonpsychopathic criminals (Group NP). Dependent variables included electrodermal responses, heart rate, respiration, and peripheral vasoconstriction. A conditioned anticipatory response (AR) was defined as a response that began between 4 and 10 seconds after CS onset; a response that began prior to this interval was considered to be an orienting response (OR) to the CS. To further reduce the effects of sensitization and pseudoconditioning, the amplitude of the AR to the CS^- was subtracted from the amplitude of the AR to the $CS^+ \text{-}S$ and the $CS^+ \text{-}P$; the results are, therefore, plotted as differential ARs.

Although the data haven't all been analyzed, the results so far are interesting. For example, Figure 7 clearly indicates that the psychopaths gave extremely small electrodermal ARs prior to shock or pictures of nude females. These results suggest that psychopaths are inferior to nonpsychopaths, not only in fear conditioning, but also (though to a lesser extent) in reward conditioning. However, this conclusion may be restricted to the use of electrodermal activity as the dependent variable. Consider Figure 8, for example, which shows conditioned finger vasoconstriction to shock and pictures. The psychopaths conditioned very well indeed and were even somewhat superior to the nonpsychopaths in both fear and reward conditioning. Similarly, psychopaths showed as much conditioned cardiac deceleration to stimuli preceding shock and pictures as did nonpsychopaths.

Whatever the interpretation of these data, it is clear that simple generalizations about the psychopath's conditionability are probably not warranted unless we are willing to restrict ourselves to electrodermal conditioning. It is possible, of course, that when noxious stimuli are involved, electrodermal activity is a better (at least simpler and clearer) indicant of fear arousal than is cardiovascular activity. While electrodermal mechanisms are innervated solely by sympathetic fibers, cardiac activity is controlled by both sympathetic and parasympathetic fibers. Further, there is a considerable

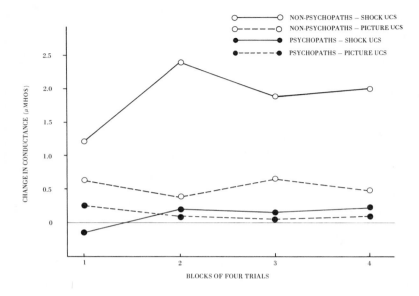

Figure 7

Differential electrodermal ARs to stimuli followed by shock and by pictures. (Modified from Quinn, 1969.)

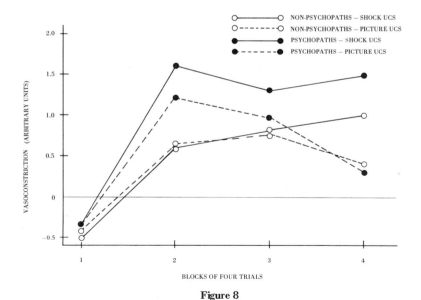

Figure 8

Differential vasomotor ARs to stimuli followed by shock and by pictures. (Modified from Quinn, 1969.)

amount of interaction between the various activities of the cardiovascular system — e.g., heart rate, blood volume, blood pressure, stroke volume, etc. — and it is, therefore, difficult to know exactly what the implications of cardiovascular conditioning are.

Avoidance learning. In his two-factor theory of avoidance learning, Mowrer (1947) postulates two stages in learning to avoid punishment. In the first stage, cues associated with punishment acquire the capacity to elicit classically conditioned fear responses. The second stage consists of the reinforcement, by fear reduction, of responses that are instrumental in removing the organism from the fear producing cues. The subject can avoid punishment by inhibiting the punished response (passive avoidance) or by making some other response (active avoidance). Concerning the former, Mowrer (1947) states:

> The performance of any given act normally produces kinesthetic (and often visual, auditory, and tactual) stimuli which are perceptible to the performer of the act. If these stimuli are followed a few times by a noxious ("unconditioned") stimulus, they will soon acquire the capacity to produce the emotion of fear. When, therefore, on subsequent occasions the subject starts to perform the previously punished act, the resulting self-stimulation will arouse fear; and the most effective way of eliminating this fear is for the subject to stop the activity which is producing the fear-producing stimuli. (p. 136)

A considerable amount of research supports this conception of acquired fear as a powerful motivator and regulator of behavior (Brown & Farber, 1968).

The relevance of two-factor theory to psychopathy is that psychopaths appear to have a low capacity for fear conditioning (at least as reflected in electrodermal activity) and they should, therefore, find it difficult to avoid punishment or to learn responses that are mediated by fear. To test this prediction in a laboratory situation, Lykken (1955) had psychopathic and neurotic criminals and normal noncriminals learn an ingeniously devised "mental maze". The apparatus was a panel on which there were four levers, a green light, a red light, and a counter labeled "errors". The subject's task was to learn a "maze" that consisted of a sequence of choices among the four levers. There were 20 points of choice and, at each point, the machine notified the subject whether he was correct. For a correct response, the green light flashed and the machine "moved," with a sound of relays operating, to the next point. At an incorrect response (any of the other three levers), the red light would flash and an error would be recorded on the counter. In addition, one of the three incorrect responses at each point was punished by a strong electric shock. Thus the subject had a twofold task. The manifest task was to make the correct responses. At the same time, he could avoid painful punishment by learning to avoid the levers that produced shock. This was the "latent" or hidden task; no mention was made of it to the subject. Each subject was given 20 trials, with the 20-choice sequence the same for each trial.

There were no differences between groups in the rate at which the manifest task was learned, indicating that maze learning ability per se was similar for each group. In order to obtain a measure of avoidance learning (latent task), the ratio of shocked to unshocked errors was computed for each subject: the lower the ratio, the greater the avoidance of shock. The results are plotted in Figure 9. It is readily apparent that both the neurotic criminals and the normal noncriminals learned to avoid shock (both groups showed a decreasing avoidance ratio), whereas the psychopaths did not. Moreover, the psychopaths had a significantly higher overall avoidance ratio than did either of the other two groups. Considered in conjunction with the already discussed studies of fear conditionability, Lykken's findings provide support for the hypothesis that psychopathy is related to poor avoidance learning. Additional support for this hypothesis has been provided by several more recent studies (Schachter & Latané, 1964; Schmauk, 1970, Schoenherr, 1964), each of which used electric shock and a "maze" similar to the one just described. In each case, psychopaths did well on the manifest task but not on the avoidance task.

If learning to avoid punishment is dependent upon the experience of anticipatory fear, it should be possible to improve the psychopath's performance by somehow augmenting his fear responses. To investigate this possibility, Schachter and Latané had their subjects learn Lykken's "maze" both with and without an injection of adrenalin, a sympathetic nervous system stimulant. The results without adrenalin were essentially the same as those reported above, i.e., psychopaths learned the manifest task, but not the latent one of avoiding shocked errors. However, when injected with adrenalin, the psychopaths did very well at avoiding shock. On the assumption that adrenalin-induced sympathetic activity augments the experience of fear, these results support the hypothesis that the psychopath's apparent inability to avoid punishment is related to inadequate anticipatory fear responses.

Adrenalin may not be the only way of increasing the psychopath's ability to avoid punishment. It is possible that stronger punishments are needed, since those generally used in these experiments may not really be painful enough either to generate anticipatory fear or to warrant special attempts to avoid them (cf. Figure 6). It is also possible that the use of punishments that are more relevant to the psychopath's value system would be more effective. Schmauk, for example, found that while psychopaths apparently made little attempt to avoid shock or social disapproval, they were quite willing and able to avoid monetary loss. It is of considerable interest here that psychopaths gave appropriate anticipatory fear (GSR) responses and were aware of the

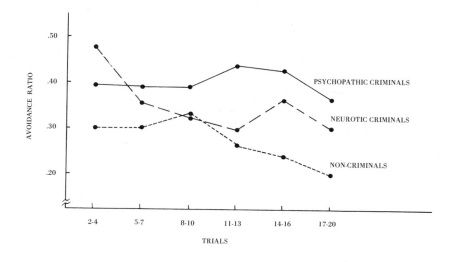

Figure 9

Avoidance ratio (shocked errors/nonshocked errors) as a function of trials.
A decreasing avoidance ratio indicates learning to avoid shocked errors.
After Lykken (1955).

contingency between their behavior and its consequences only when the
punishment involved was loss of money.

Anticipation of Punishment

I have suggested that the psychopath's relative inability to avoid
punishment is related to the failure of cues associated with punishment to
elicit sufficient anticipatory fear for the instigation and subsequent reinforcement of avoidance responses. In a social context, ability to inhibit responses
that have previously been punished may be analogous to the concept of
conscience or, more specifically, to resistance to temptation. Note that the
cues eliciting fear may be symbolic or verbal in nature. For example, the
psychopathic person may say to himself, "If I do this, I may get caught and
be punished." However, these cues are presumably devoid of appropriate
emotional content, a situation very similar to Cleckley's concept of semantic
dementia. To put it another way, the psychopath does not anticipate, in an
emotional sense, the unpleasant consequences of his own behavior. In general,
the normal individual's anticipation of pain or discomfort is what Freud
(1936) referred to as *objective anxiety or fear* — an emotional state triggered

31

off by danger signals and characterized by feelings of apprehension and autonomic arousal. According to Freud, a strong anxiety response motivates the individual to remove himself from the source of danger, a concept not unlike Mowrer's two-factor theory. It is obvious that objective anxieties (Freud) or conditioned anticipatory fear responses (Mowrer) have a considerable amount of functional significance for the normal individual.

We might assume that the degree of apprehension, anxiety, or fear experienced by an individual is inversely related to the remoteness in time of the anticipated pain or discomfort. That is, an aversive event anticipated in the very near future is more fear arousing than a similar event more remote in time (see Figure 10). This hypothesis is based on the assumption that the degree of fear elicited by cues associated with impending or threatened punishment is directly related to the salience of these cues, and that their salience decreases with increased temporal remoteness. There are several reasons for hypothesizing that this *temporal gradient* of fear arousal is steeper for psychopaths than for normal persons. For example, one of the striking things about the psychopath is what has been termed his "short-range hedonism" (Hare, 1965a) — a tendency to satisfy immediate needs even at the risk of experiencing severe discomfort in the future. This suggests that future pain and discomfort are of little immediate consequence to him. Further, it is possible to conceive of a temporal gradient of fear arousal as a form of stimulus generalization in which the stimulus dimension is a temporal one. Since psychopaths show less generalization of a conditioned fear response than do normal persons (Hare, 1965b), at least when the stimulus dimension is physical similarity, they should, by implication, also show less temporal generalization. Moreover, as Figure 10 indicates, their temporal gradient of fear arousal should be lower in height than that of other individuals, since their acquired fear responses are relatively small (Lykken, 1955; Quinn, 1969). Some empirical support for these temporal gradients has been provided by several recent studies. In one study (Hare, 1965c), subjects watched consecutive numbers, 1-12, appear in the window of a memory drum. After this first trial, each subject was told that the series of numbers would be repeated several times and that each time the number eight appeared, he would receive an electric shock equal in intensity to one earlier determined to be the strongest he could tolerate. Skin conductance was monitored throughout the six trials given. During the first trial (nonshock), all subjects showed a gradual decrease in skin conductance. The results for Trials 2 and 6 (first and last shock trials) are plotted in Figure 11. Compared to the nonpsychopathic criminals (NP) and noncriminal subjects (C), the psychopathic criminals (P) showed very little anticipatory GSR activity prior to the advent of shock. To the extent that skin conductance increases can be considered an indicant of fear arousal, these results suggest that, unless the

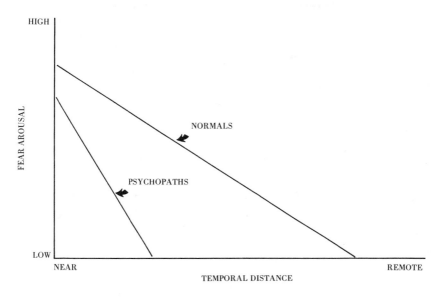

Figure 10

Hypothetical relationship between fear arousal and the temporal remoteness of anticipated pain or punishment. After Hare (1965a), *J. of Research in Crime and Delinquency*. Reprinted with permission of National Council on Crime and Delinquency.

cues are in close temporal proximity to punishment, they elicit very little fear in the psychopath; i.e. he has a steep temporal gradient of fear arousal.

Somewhat similar results were obtained by Lippert and Senter (1966). Their subjects were told that at the end of a 10-minute period (a clock was visible) they would receive a strong electric shock through electrodes attached to the leg. During this period, the nonpsychopathic subjects showed a considerably greater increase in spontaneous GSR activity than did the psychopathic subjects. Moreover, just before the shock was due, the nonpsychopaths displayed a sharp increase in skin conductance, while none of the psychopaths did so. It is worthwhile noting here that shock was not actually administered at any time during the experiment, so that the results are not due to any group differences in sensitivity to shock. In a recent study, Schalling and Levander (1967) also found that psychopathic delinquents showed less anticipatory spontaneous GSR activity before shock than did anxious delinquents.

The hypothesis that psychopaths have a steeper-than-normal temporal gradient of fear arousal has been incorporated (Hare, 1965a) into a simple model of psychopathy based upon Miller's (1959) well-known approach-

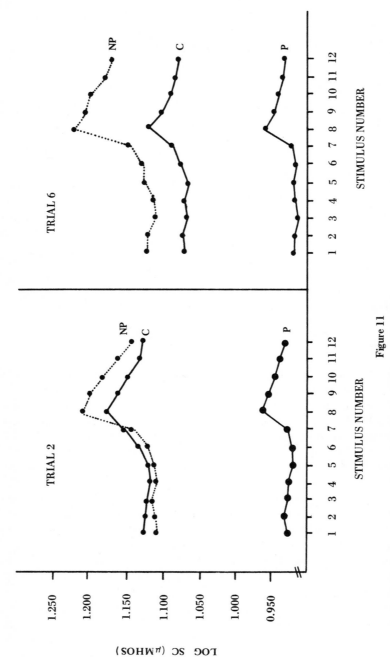

Figure 11

Log conductance level as a function of anticipated shock (administered at stimulus number 8). P = psychopathic criminals; NP = nonpsychopathic criminals; C = normal noncriminals. From Hare (1965c), *J. Abnorm. Psychol.*, 70, 442-445. Reprinted with permission of American Psychological Association.

avoidance theory of behavior. The model is based upon the assumption that the tendency to avoid or inhibit a punished response is a function of the degree of conditioned fear elicited by cues associated with the response. Viewed in this way, Figure 10 can also represent the tendency to avoid or inhibit responses as a function of the temporal interval between the response and the anticipated punishment. For instance, all other things being equal, a psychopath would be less likely than would a normal person to inhibit a response, regardless of whether punishment is expected immediately or in the future. It is obvious, of course, that expectation of punishment is not the only factor determining whether some specific behavior will occur. Many responses, for example, are ambivalent in nature, having both positive (rewarding) and negative (punishing) consequences. In effect, the individual is motivated to make the response and, at the same time, to inhibit it. Whether the response occurs, then, depends upon the relative weights assigned by the individual to the positive and negative consequences of the response. However, the individual's task is complicated by the fact that the anticipated rewards and punishments are located at different points in time. Thus a response may have immediate rewarding features but delayed unpleasant consequences, and vice versa. The individual's task is, therefore, one of *temporal integration* (Renner, 1964) in which the relative value or utility of reward and punishment, and hence the relative tendency to make or inhibit a response is a function of their temporal distance from the response.

By combining the gradients in Figure 10 with postulated temporal reward gradients, we arrive at Figure 12. Originally (Hare, 1965a), I had assumed that temporal reward gradients were the same for both psychopaths and normal individuals, largely because relevant data were absent. However, I think that on the basis of Quinn's (1969) study, as well as what we know of psychopaths clinically, a more reasonable assumption is that their temporal reward gradient, like their temporal gradient of fear arousal and response inhibition, is lower and steeper than it is for normal persons — that is, neither reward nor punishments exist for the psychopath when they are too far in the future.

With the baseline in Figure 12 representing the estimated time between an action and its consequences, it is evident that if the positive and negative consequences are both expected in the immediate future (e.g., at time A), both psychopaths and normal persons would avoid the action, since the tendency to inhibit the response is greater than the tendency to make it. On the other hand, if the positive consequences are expected at time A and the negative consequences at a later time (e.g., at time B), then the normal person, but not the psychopath, would inhibit the response, since the tendency to inhibit the response is greater than the tendency to make it for the normal person but not for the psychopath. Of course, if the negative consequences are very remote (e.g., at time C), then even the normal person

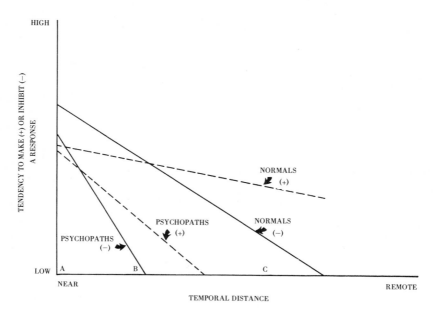

Figure 12

The postulated tendency to make or inhibit a response as a function of the temporal remoteness of anticipated reward and punishment. From Hare (1965a), *J. of Research in Crime and Delinquency*. Reprinted with permission of National Council on Crime and Delinquency.

would make the response. In many ways, this latter situation is analogous with the "live now — pay later" approach to life that is not uncommon in our society. (For the psychopath, the philosophy is more likely to be "live now — pay never.")

The model outlined in Figure 12 would predict that deferred payments (negative consequences) and immediate enjoyment (positive consequences) are even more attractive to the psychopath than to the normal person; the psychopath should be (and is) constantly in trouble with credit agencies and finance companies. Moreover, the fact that many psychopaths have a penchant for cashing bad checks and fraudulently obtaining goods is consistent with the model, since immediate rewards more than offset the possible effects of future punishments.[8]

---

[8]Noting that the psychopath does not experience the sort of anxiety associated with future punishment, Arieti (1967) states that, "He knows theoretically that he may be caught in the antisocial act and be punished. But again, this punishment is a possibility concerning the future and, therefore, he does not experience the idea of it with enough emotional strength to change the course of his present actions." (p. 248)

The baseline in Figures 10 and 12 can also be representative of other dimensions, including spatial distance from a goal and similarities between situations and actions. For example, if the baseline in Figure 12 represents similarity between different social situations, we would expect that the effect of punishing the psychopath in one situation would not generalize to other situations unless they were highly similar to the original one. The normal person, on the other hand, would tend to inhibit behavior in a wide variety of situations similar to the one in which the behavior was actually punished. If we assume that the process of socialization involves not only learning to inhibit certain responses, but also the generalization of these inhibitory tendencies to other relevant situations, the model would predict poorer socialization in the psychopath than in the normal individual.

Cleckley (1964) has described the psychopath as an individual whose verbalizations (e.g., "I'm really sorry for what I did") appear normal but are devoid of the appropriate emotional content, a disorder that he has termed *semantic dementia*. As Johns and Quay (1962) have put it, the psychopath knows the words but not the music. I think that this whole concept of semantic dementia is worth investigating thoroughly, and that it could be cast into terms that are familiar to the experimental psychologist. For example, it is quite possible that semantic dementia represents the failure of emotional responses that have been conditioned to one word to generalize to other similar words; that is, the psychopath may show little semantic generalization of emotional responses, or, as the Russians put it, little generalization within the second signaling system. To investigate this possibility, we are currently planning an experiment in which psychopaths and normal individuals will be compared on the generalization of autonomic, skeletal-muscular, and meaning responses across semantic and physical dimensions (the latter representing generalization within the first signaling system).

Perhaps related to the concept of semantic dementia is the assumption that the psychopath is unable to experience the emotional correlates of empathy, although he may verbally express concern for the distress and misfortunes of others. Ax (1962) has suggested that empathy and the accurate perception of another's feelings and attitudes may require the construction of an "emotional facsimile" involving the higher centers of the autonomic nervous system. If these centers are preoccupied with other processes, such as hostility or activity concerned with the self, or if they do not function properly, they may be unable to create the "empathic hypotheses" needed to simulate another's feelings. The implication here is that the psychopath's lack of empathy may be associated with the failure (or inability) to give the appropriate autonomic responses to the suffering and distress of others and to situations involving the interpersonal exchange of love, affection, remorse, etc. To investigate this possibility, we are conducting an experiment in which subjects are required to administer shocks, under

37

various conditions, to a "stooge" who has the opportunity of retaliating. Our prediction is that the psychopath will verbally express concern and distress over the suffering of the other person, but that the appropriate autonomic correlates will be absent. We are also interested in whether the psychopath is capable of vicarious conditioning to the cues associated with the rewards and punishments administered to others (cf. Craig & Lowery, 1969). If he is incapable of acquiring conditioned responses vicariously, an important means of obtaining information about the contingencies in his environment (observational learning, modeling, role-playing, etc.) would largely be denied him.

As a final comment, I should note that although the gradient model outlined above is primarily a conditioning one, it is possible to relate it to subcortical mechanisms in the brain. Stein (1964), for example, has proposed that it is the anticipation or expectation of rewards and punishments, not their actual occurrence, that motivates behavior. He also argues that the mechanism for reinforcement is a classically conditioned anticipatory response that activates either reward or punishment mechanisms in the hypothalamus, thereby facilitating or inhibiting ongoing behavior. By the same token, the psychopath's low capacity for fear (and reward?) conditioning could mean that the expectation of future rewards and punishments does not activate the appropriate subcortical mechanisms and, therefore, has little effect upon his immediate behavior. Other cortical mechanisms may also be involved in the psychopath's failure to anticipate events in the environment. W. Grey Walter (1964), for example, has found that the expectancy that some significant event will occur is associated with a slow increase in the negative potential of the frontal cortex. Walter refers to this change as the *contingent negative variation* (CNV) or *expectancy wave*, and McCallum (1967) reports that it is absent in psychopaths.

References

Albert, R. S., Brigante, T. R., & Chase, M. The psychopathic personality: A content analysis of the concept. *Journal of General Psychology*, 1959, **60**, 17-28.

Alexander, F. The neurotic character. *International Journal of Psychoanalysis*, 1930, **11**, 292-311.

American Psychiatric Association. *Diagnostic and statistical manual: Mental disorders*. Washington, D.C.: Author, 1952.

Arieti, S. *The intrapsychic self*. New York: Basic Books, 1967.

Ax, A. F. Psychophysiological methodology for the study of schizophrenia. In R. Ressler & N. Greenfield (Eds.), *Physiological correlates of psychological disorder*. Madison: University of Wisconsin Press, 1962. Pp. 29-44.

Bay-Rakal, S. The significance of EEG abnormality in behaviour problem children. *Canadian Psychiatric Association Journal*, 1965, **10**, 387-91.

Bernard, J. L. & Eisenman, R. Verbal conditioning in sociopaths with social and monetary reinforcement. *Journal of Personality and Social Psychology*, 1967, **6**, 203-06.

Blaylock, J. J. Verbal conditioning performance of psychopaths and nonpsychopaths under verbal reward and punishment. Unpublished doctoral dissertation, State University of Iowa, 1960.

Brown, J. S. & Farber, I. E. Secondary motivational systems. In P. R. Farnsworth (Ed.), *Annual Review of Psychology*. Vol. 19, Palo Alto: Annual Review, 1968. Pp. 99-134.

Bryan, J. H. & Kapche, R. Psychopathy and verbal conditioning. *Journal of Abnormal Psychology*, 1967, **72**, 71-73.

Cleckley, H. *The mask of sanity*. (4th ed.) St. Louis, Mo.: Mosby, 1964.

Craddick, R. A. Wechsler-Bellevue, I.Q. scores of psychopathic and nonpsychopathic prisoners. *Journal of Psychological Studies*, 1961, **12**, 167-72.

Craft, M. J. *Ten studies into psychopathic personality*. Bristol: John Wright, 1965.

Craig, K. & Lowery, J. Heart rate components of conditioned vicarious autonomic responses. *Journal of Personality and Social Psychology*, 1969, **11**, 381-87.

Currie, J. S. *Performance of sociopaths, anxiety neurotics and normals on a complex perceptual task under conditions of limited exposure duration.* (Doctoral dissertation, University of Florida) Ann Arbor, Mich.: University Microfilms, 1965. No. 66-2015.

Dain, N. & Carlson, F. Moral insanity in the United States 1835-66. *American Journal of Psychology*, 1962, **118**, 795-800.

Douglas, R. J. The hippocampus and behaviour. *Psychological Bulletin*, 1967, **67**, 416-42.

Eysenck, H. J. *The biological basis of personality.* Springfield, Ill.: Charles C. Thomas, 1967.

Fairweather, G. W. The effect of selected incentive conditions on the performance of psychopathic, neurotic, and normal criminals in a serial rote learning situation. Unpublished doctoral dissertation, University of Illinois, 1953.

Finney, J. C. Relations and meaning of the new MMPI scales. *Psychological Reports*, 1966, **18**, 459-70.

Forssman, H. & Frey, T. S. Electroencephalograms of boys with behaviour disorders. *Acta Psychiatrica Neurologica Scandinavica*, 1953, **28**, 61-73.

Fox, R. & Lippert, W. Spontaneous GSR and anxiety level in sociopathic delinquents. *Journal of Consulting Psychology*, 1963, **27**, 368.

Freud, S. *The problem of anxiety.* New York: Norton, 1936.

Gellhorn, E. *Autonomic imbalance and the hypothalamus: Implications for physiology, medicine, psychology, and neuropsychiatry.* Minneapolis: University of Minnesota Press, 1957.

Goldstein, I. B. The relationship of muscle tension and autonomic activity to psychiatric disorders. *Psychosomatic Medicine*, 1965, **27**, 39-52.

Gray, K. C. & Hutchison, H. C. The psychopathic personality: A survey of Canadian psychiatrists' opinions. *Canadian Psychiatric Association Journal*, 1964, **9**, 452-61.

Grossman, S. B. *A textbook of physiological psychology.* New York: Wiley, 1967.

Group for the Advancement of Psychiatry. *Psychopathological disorders in children: Theoretical considerations and a proposed classification.* Report No. 62. New York: Author, 1966.

Gurvitz, M. Wechsler-Bellevue test and the diagnosis of psychopathic personality. *Journal of Clinical Psychology*, 1950, **6**, 397-401.

Hare, R. D. A conflict and learning theory analysis of psychopathic behaviour. *Journal of Research in Crime and Delinquency*, 1965, **2**, 12-19. (a)

Hare, R. D. Acquisition and generalization of a conditioned-fear response in psychopathic and nonpsychopathic criminals. *Journal of Psychology*, 1965, **59**, 367-70. (b)

Hare, R. D. Temporal gradient of fear arousal in psychopaths. *Journal of Abnormal Psychology*, 1965, **70**, 442-45. (c)

Hare, R. D. Psychopathy fear arousal and anticipated pain. *Psychological Reports*, 1965, **16**, 499-502. (d)

Hare, R. D. Psychopathy and choice of immediate versus delayed punishment. *Journal of Abnormal Psychology*, 1966, **71**, 25-29. (a)

Hare, R. D. Psychopathy, autonomic functioning, and the orienting response. *Journal of Abnormal Psychology*, 1968, **73**, (3, Pt. 2), 1-24. (a)

Hare, R. D. Detection threshold for electric shock in psychopaths. *Journal of Abnormal Psychology*, 1968, **73**, 268-72. (b)

Hare, R. D. *Psychopathy: Theory and research*. New York: Wiley, 1970.

Hare, R. D. & Hare, A. S. Psychopathic behaviour: A bibliography. *Excerpta Criminologica*, 1967, **7**, 365-86.

Hare, R. D. & Thorvaldson, S. A. Psychopathy and sensitivity to electrical stimulation. *Journal of Abnormal Psychology*, 1970, **76**, 370-74.

Harter, M. R. Excitability cycles and cortical scanning: A review of two hypotheses of central intermittency in perception. *Psychological Bulletin*, 1967, **68**, 47-58.

Hill, D. EEG in episodic psychotic and psychopathic behaviour: A classification of data. *EEG and Clinical Neurophysiology*, 1952, 4, 419-42.

Hughes, J. R. A review of the positive spike phenomenon. In W. Wilson (Ed.), *Applications of electroencephalography in psychiatry*. Durham, N.C.: Duke University Press, 1965. Pp. 54-101.

Jenkins, R. L. Diagnosis, dynamics and treatment in child psychiatry. *Psychiatric Research Reports*, 1964, **18**, 91-120.

Jenkins, R. L. Psychiatric syndromes in children and their relation to family background. *American Journal of Orthopsychiatry*, 1966, **36**, 450-57.

Johns, J. H. & Quay, H. C. The effect of social reward on verbal conditioning in psychopathic and neurotic military offenders. *Journal of Consulting Psychology*, 1962, **26**, 217-20.

Kadlub, K. J. The effects of two types of reinforcements on the performance of psychopathic and normal criminals. Unpublished doctoral dissertation, University of Illinois, 1956.

Karpman, B. The structure of neurosis: With special differentials between neurosis, psychosis, homosexuality, alcoholism, psychopathy, and criminality. *Archives of Criminal Psychodynamics*, 1961, 4, 599-646.

Kiloh, L. & Osselton, J. W. *Clinical electroencephalography*. Washington: Butterworth, 1966.

Kimble, G. Categories of learning and the problem of definition. In A. W. Melton (Ed.), *Categories of human learning*. New York: Academic Press, 1964. Pp. 34-45.

Kimmel, H. D. Inhibition of the unconditioned response in classical conditioning. *Psychological Review*, 1966, 73, 232-40.

Kurland, H. D., Yeager, C. T., & Arthur, R. J. Psychophysiologic aspects of severe behaviour disorders. *Archives of General Psychiatry*, 1963, 8, 599-604.

Lacey, J. I. Somatic response patterning and stress: Some revisions of activation theory. In M. H. Appley & R. Trumbell (Eds.), *Psychological stress: Issues in research*. New York: Appleton-Century-Crofts, 1967. Pp. 14-44.

Lacey, J. I. & Lacey, B. C. The relationship of resting autonomic activity to motor impulsivity. In *The brain and human behaviour* (Proceedings of the Association for Research in Neural and Mental Disease). Baltimore: William & Wilkins, 1958. Pp. 144-209.

Lindner, R. Experimental studies in constitutional psychopathic inferiority. Part 1. Systemic patterns. *Journal of Criminal Psychopathology*, 1942, 3, 252-76.

Lindsley, D. B. The ontogeny of pleasure: Neural and behavioural development. In R. G. Heath (Ed.), *The role of pleasure in behaviour*. New York: Harper & Row, 1964. Pp. 3-22.

Lippert, W. W. & Senter, R. J. Electrodermal responses in the sociopath. *Psychonomic Science*, 1966, 4, 25-26.

Lykken, D. T. *A study of anxiety in the sociopathic personality*. (Doctoral dissertation, University of Minnesota) Ann Arbor, Mich.: University Microfilms, 1955. No. 55-944.

Lynn, R. *Attention, arousal, and the orientation reaction*. London: Pergamon Press, 1966.

Malmo, R. B. Studies of anxiety: Some clinical origins of the activation concept. In C. D. Spielberger (Ed.), *Anxiety and behaviour*. New York: Academic Press, 1966. Pp. 157-78.

Maughs, S. B. Concept of psychopathy and psychopathic personality: Its evolution and historical development. *Journal of Criminal Psychopathology*, 1941, 2, 329-56, 365-99.

McCallum, C. The contingent negative variation. Unpublished doctoral dissertation, University of Bristol, 1967.

McCleary, R. A. Response-modulating functions of the limbic system: Initiation and suppression. In E. Steller & J. Sprague (Eds.), *Progress in physiological psychology*. Vol. 1. New York: Academic Press, 1966. Pp. 209-72.

McCord, W. & McCord, J. *The psychopath: An essay on the criminal mind.* Princeton: Van Nostrand, 1964.

McDonald, D. C., Johnson, L. C., & Hord, D. J. Habituation of the orienting response in alert and drowsy subjects. *Psychophysiology*, 1964, 1, 163-73.

Miller, J. G. *Eyeblink conditioning of primary and neurotic psychopaths.* (Doctoral dissertation, University of Missouri) Ann Arbor, Mich.: University Microfilms, 1966. No. 67-923.

Miller, N. E. Liberalization of basic S-R concepts: Extensions to conflict behaviour, motivation and social learning. In S. Koch (Ed.), *Psychology: A study of a science*. Vol. 2. New York: McGraw-Hill, 1959.

Mowrer, O. H. On the dual nature of learning — a reinterpretation of "conditioning" and "problem-solving". *Harvard Educational Review*, 1947, 17, 102-48.

Orris, J. B. Visual monitoring performance in three subgroups of male delinquents. Unpublished master's thesis, University of Illinois, 1967.

Painting, D. H. The performance of psychopathic individuals under conditions of positive and negative partial reinforcement. *Journal of Abnormal and Social Psychology*, 1961, 62, 352-55.

Peterson, D. R., Quay, H. C., & Tiffany, T. L. Personality factors related to juvenile delinquency. *Child Development*, 1961, 32, 355-72.

Petrie, A. *Individuality in pain and suffering.* Chicago: University of Chicago Press, 1967.

Phillips, L. A social view of psychopathology. In P. London & D. Rosenhan (Eds.), *Foundations of abnormal psychology*. New York: Holt, Rinehart & Winston, 1968. Pp. 427-59.

Pribram, K. H. Emotion: Toward a neuropsychological theory. In D. C. Glass (Ed.), *Neurophysiology and emotion*. New York: Rockefeller University Press, 1967. Pp. 3-40.

Pritchard, J. *A treatise on insanity*. Philadelphia: Haswell, Barrington & Haswell, 1835.

Quay, H. C. Dimensions of personality in delinquent boys as inferred from the factor analysis of case history data. *Child Development*, 1964, 35, 479-84. (a)

Quay, H. C. Personality dimensions in delinquent males as inferred from the factor analysis of behaviour rating. *Journal of Research in Crime and Delinquency*, 1964, 1, 35-37. (b)

Quay, H. C. Psychopathic personality as pathological stimulation seeking. *American Journal of Psychiatry*, 1965, 122, 180-83.

Quay, H. C. & Hunt, W. A. Psychopathy, neuroticism and verbal conditioning: A replication and extension. *Journal of Consulting Psychology*, 1965, 29, 283.

Quinn, M. J. Psychopathy and autonomic conditioning. Unpublished doctoral dissertation, University of British Columbia, 1969.

Renner, K. E. Conflict resolution and the process of temporal integration. *Psychological Reports*, 1964, 15, (No. 2), 423-38.

Robins, Lee N. *Deviant children grown up*. Baltimore: Williams & Wilkins, 1966.

Rose, R. J. Preliminary study of three indicants of arousal: Measurement, interrelationships, and clinical correlates. Unpublished doctoral dissertation, University of Minnesota, 1964.

Ruilmann, C. J. & Gulo, M. J. Investigation of autonomic responses in psychopathic personalities. *Southern Medical Journal*, 1950, 43, 953-56.

Schachter, S. & Latane, B. Crime, cognition and the autonomic nervous system. In M. R. Jones (Ed.), *Nebraska symposium on motivation*. Lincoln: University of Nebraska Press, 1964. Pp. 221-75.

Schalling, D. & Levander, S. Rating of anxiety proneness and responses to electrical pain stimulation. *Scandinavian Journal of Psychology*, 1964, 5, 1-9.

Schalling, D. & Levander, S. Spontaneous fluctuations in EDA during anticipation of pain in two delinquent groups differing in anxiety proneness. Report No. 238 from the Psychological Laboratory, University of Stockholm, 1967.

Schalling, D., Lidberg, L., Levander, S., & Dahlin, Y. Relations between fluctuations in skin resistance and digital pulse volume and scores on the Gough De scale. Unpublished manuscript, University of Stockholm, 1968.

Scheibel, M. E. & Scheibel, A. B. Some neural substrates of postnatal development. In M. Hoffman & L. Hoffman (Eds.), *Review of child development research*. Vol. 1. New York: Russell Sage Foundation, 1954. Pp. 481-519.

Schmauk, F. J. A study of the relationship between kinds of punishment, autonomic arousal, subjective anxiety and avoidance learning in the primary sociopath. *Journal of Abnormal Psychology*, 1970, **76**, 325-55.

Schoenherr, J. C. *Avoidance of noxious stimulation in psychopathic personality*. (Doctoral dissertation, University of California, Los Angeles) Ann Arbor, Mich.: University Microfilms, 1964, No. 64-8334.

Schoper, C. A. A study of learning and retention with neutral and social-primitive words in normal, psychopathic and psychoneurotic criminals. Unpublished doctoral dissertation, University of Illinois, 1958.

Schwade, E. D. & Geiger, S. G. Abnormal electroencephalographic findings in severe behaviour disorders. *Diseases of the Nervous System*, 1965, **17**, 307-17.

Shagass, C. & Schwartz, M. Observations on somatosensory cortical reactivity in personality disorders. *Journal of Nervous and Mental Disease*, 1962, **135**, 44-51.

Sherman, L. J. Retention in psychopathic, neurotic and normal subjects. *Journal of Personality*, 1957, **6**, 722-29.

Singer, J. L. *Daydreaming*. New York: Random House, 1966.

Skrzypek, G. J. The effects of perceptual isolation and arousal on anxiety, complexity preference and novelty preference in psychopathic and neurotic delinquents. *Journal of Abnormal Psychology*, 1969, **74**, 321-29.

Sokolov, E. N. *Perception and the conditioned reflex*. New York: MacMillan, 1963.

Stein, L. Reciprocal action of reward and punishment mechanisms. In R. Heath (Ed.), *The role of pleasure in behaviour*. New York: Harper & Row, 1964. Pp. 113-39.

Stern, J. A. & McDonald, D. C. Physiological correlates of mental disease. In P. R. Farnsworth (Ed.), *Annual Review of Psychology*. Palo Alto: Annual Review, 1965. Pp. 225-64.

Tong, J. E. Stress reactivity in relation to delinquent and psychopathic behaviour. *Journal of Mental Science*, 1959, **105**, 935-56.

Walter, W. Grey. Slow potential waves in the human brain associated with expectancy, attention and decision. *Archiv für Psychiatric und Zeitschrift f.d. ges Neurologie*, 1964, **206**, 309-22.

Warren, A. B. & Grant, D. A. The relation of conditioned discrimination to MMPI Pd personality variable. *Journal of Experimental Psychology*, 1955, 49, 23-27.

Weisen, A. E. *Differential reinforcing effects of onset and offset of stimulation on the operant behaviour of normals, neurotics and psychopaths.* (Doctoral dissertation, University of Florida) Ann Arbor, Mich.: University Microfilms, 1965. No. 65-9625.

Zubin, J. Classification of the behaviour disorders. In P. R. Farnsworth (Ed.), *Annual review of psychology*. Palo Alto: Annual Reviews, 1967. Pp. 373-406.

Chapter 2

The Retarded Child as a Whole Person[1]

Edward Zigler[2]

We are presently witnessing a productive, disputatious, exciting, and perhaps inevitably chaotic period in the history of one of man's oldest and most pressing problems: mental retardation. Given the current plethora of far from consistent research reports, views, and counterviews in this area, it behooves us to anchor this particular presentation on some bedrock view to which all current thinkers could subscribe. I think that we can all agree that the essential defining feature of mental retardation is lower intelligence than that displayed by the modal member of an appropriate reference group. Stated somewhat differently, I do not believe that anyone would argue with the statement that a seven-year-old retarded child is less intelligent than a seven-year-old child of average intellect. Unfortunately, when we venture even a short distance from this statement, we immediately find ourselves adrift on a sea of definitional uncertainty. For, if we ask the rather basic question of what we mean by intelligence, we quickly encounter considerable disagreement.

Many insist that intelligence refers to nothing more than the quality of the behaviors emitted by the individual assessed against some criterion of social competence. Others have argued that a clear distinction must be drawn between intelligence and the sheer manifestation of adaptive or socially competent behaviors which are typically labeled "intelligent." Inherent in this latter position is the view that behaviors indicative of social competence do not inevitably reflect normal intellectual functioning anymore than the relative absence of such behaviors in the emotionally unstable, the criminal, or the social misfit inevitably reflects intellectual subnormality. Thinkers who

[1]I would like to dedicate this paper to the memory of Ida Axelrod of the National Association for Retarded Children. As a result of her untimely death, we have lost a wonderful person devoted to the betterment of the lives of the retarded through research.

[2]The preparation of this paper was facilitated by Research Grant HD-03008 from the United States Public Health Service, and by the Gunnar Dybwad Award of the National Association for Retarded Children. The author is indebted to Susan Harter, David Balla, and Thomas Achenbach for their critical reading of this paper.

have espoused this latter view, including myself, have argued that the concept of social competence is much too vague and that the behaviors, often placed within its rubric, frequently partake of nonintellective influences. As a result, they have concluded that the ultimate referents of intelligence cannot be the sheer manifestation or nonmanifestation of a wide variety of behaviors that are rather arbitrarily designated as socially competent.

However, in seeking some more satisfying definition of intelligence, this group, too, has been rather arbitrary. I am very much afraid that definition making is inevitably arbitrary and that, therefore, it is fruitless to argue whether a definition is true or false. The more appropriate point of contention is whether one definition is more useful than another in respect to organizing our thinking, bringing clarity to areas of confusion, and more usefully giving direction to our empirical efforts. With such criteria in mind, I, along with others, have argued that intelligence is a hypothetical construct having, as its ultimate referents, the cognitive processes of the individual, e.g., thought, memory, concept formation, and reasoning. Approached in this way, the problem of defining intelligence becomes one with the problem of the nature of cognition and its development. On this point, I am in agreement with Tuddenham (1962) who has noted that a theory of intelligence must provide an explanation of the curve of change in cognitive ability throughout the entire life span, must deal with the ontogenesis of the psychological processes which mediate test performance, and must encompass the organization and vicissitudes of these processes from earliest infancy to senescence.

The delineation of cognition and its development as the essential focus of intelligence, and thus of mental retardation, has a certain appeal since it relates so readily to at least one easily observable phenomenon that forever differentiates the retarded individual from one of average intellect. Two individuals of quite disparate IQs, for example, one of 70 and one of 100, may be employed at the same occupation, be members of the same union, participate in the same type of community and recreational activities, and may be both successfully married and raising a family. From the viewpoint of standard social competence indices, these two individuals appear to be quite similar. However, when we shift our attention from such social competence indices to the development and present manifestation of the formal cognitive characteristics of these two individuals, we have no difficulty distinguishing between them. They function quite differently on a wide variety of cognitive tasks, devised by such cognitive theorists as Bartlett, Bruner, Ebbinghaus, Piaget, and Vygotsky, as well as across a wide array of tests employed by such psychometricians as Binet and Wechsler, tests which also assess, albeit far from perfectly, basic cognitive processes. When examined in adulthood, the individual of 100 IQ is superior to the individual of 70 IQ in meeting the cognitive demands posed by these tasks. Thus we do little injustice if we say that, at the peak of their intellectual functioning, the cognitive functioning of the individual of average intellect is at a higher level than is that of the retarded individual.

If we approach the cognitive differences between these two individuals from a developmental point of view, as Piaget and the Geneva group have done (Inhelder, 1968), we can observe that the retarded individual progresses through the same sequence of early stages of cognitive development as does the individual of average intellect, but the retarded individual does so at a slower rate. It would thus appear that the essential difference between the retarded individual and the individual of average intellect is a difference in the rate of cognitive development as well as in the ultimate or final level of cognition achieved. At any particular stage of development, the individual's cognitive level is comprised of the sum total of cognitive processes. This collection of processes thus constitutes the information processing system which mediates both inputs from the environment and responses that the individual makes in his efforts after adaptation. It is clear that the quality or nature of this information processing system must have profound and pervasive effects on the individual's behavior.

With the exception of my more radically empirical friends in the behavior modification area who would argue against both this cognitive emphasis and the need for a human typology which includes individuals of retarded, normal, and superior intellect, many thinkers would agree that it is only through reference to differences in the development and final level of formal cognitive functioning that the distinction between the intellectually retarded and the nonretarded can be reliably and consistently drawn.

Now that we have constructed a reasonable and, in my opinion, valid frame of reference concerning the essential differences between the intellectually retarded and the nonretarded, it becomes my task to convince you that overemphasizing this basically sound position has resulted, at best, in incomplete and, at worst, totally erroneous explanations as to why, in prescribed situations, the retarded behave as they do. Let me be clear on this matter. As stated above, the cognitive functioning of the retarded, which is poorer in quality than that of the individual of average intellect, has a profound and pervasive influence on his general behavior. The crucial questions here are: just how profound and just how pervasive is this influence, and how does this influence vary across tasks with which the retarded is confronted? What must be grasped is that the behavior of the retarded, as for all human beings, reflects more than the formal cognitive processes that we have been discussing up to this point.

Since there is considerable agreement that a deficiency in cognitive functioning is the essential defining feature of mental retardation, it is easy to see why workers have concentrated on cognitive determinants and have underemphasized, if not almost totally excluded, other factors influencing the behavior of the retarded. There is clearly a tendency to attribute all of the atypical behavior of the retarded to their cognitive deficiency. We appear to be so awed with the cognitive shortcomings of the retarded that we are led into tautologies in which we assert that retarded individuals behave the way they do because they are retarded. More sophisticated theoretical efforts have attempted to avoid this circularity, attributing behavioral differences between retarded and normal individuals, not to the global phenomenon of mental retardation, but rather to some specific hypothesized defect or behavioral deficiency thought to characterize intellectually retarded functioning. Thus, over the years, we have been informed that the retarded suffer from a relative impermeability of the boundaries between regions in the cognitive structure (Kounin, 1941a,b; Lewin, 1936), primary and secondary rigidity caused by subcortical and cortical malformations, respectively (Goldstein, 1943), inadequate neural satiation related to brain modifiability or cortical conductivity (Spitz, 1963), impaired attention directing mechanisms (Zeaman, 1959), a relative brevity in the persistence of stimulus trace (Siegel & Foshee, 1960), and improper development of the verbal systems resulting in a dissociation between the verbal and motor systems (Luria, 1956; O'Connor & Hermelin, 1959).

Included in this list are concepts which lie at the center of some of the most important programmatic theoretical efforts in the area of mental retardation. The adversarial stance that I have taken over the years toward the need to invoke such concepts when explaining differences in behavior between groups of MA-matched, familial retardeds and normals is by now well-known. However, I have also gone on record as believing that these theoretical formulations are viable ones and are unquestionably valuable in that they lead us away from a rather sterile global approach toward a more fine-grained analysis of the cognitive processes of both retarded and normal individuals. In noting the cognitive deficiencies listed above, we need not become bogged down in the developmental versus difference controversy over the nature of mental retardation, about which I have written at some length. A listing of these positions is relevant to this presentation only to the extent that it reflects the fact that the bulk of theoretical and empirical efforts in the area of mental retardation is concerned with the cognitive shortcomings of the retarded individual. As this list of cognitive deficiencies, from which the retarded are thought to suffer, has grown over the years, it has become an increasingly simple matter to explain any and all differences in behavior between normal and retarded individuals with the *post hoc* selection from this list of a factor which appears even remotely relevant to the behavioral differences in question. Having been misinterpreted in the past, I want to be perfectly clear here. My statement is in no way an indictment of the theoretician who is carefully exploring the cognitive variable that interests him. It is an indictment of the after-the-fact "theorizing" which allows the thinker to evade any real coming to grips with the complexities of his subject matter.

While no exception can be taken to circumscribed cognitive hypotheses concerning mental retardation, I must assert again that any cognitive theory cannot be a complete theory of the behavior of the retarded since the behavior of the retarded, like that of any other group of humans, reflects factors other than cognitive ones. While the analogy is far from perfect, it should be noted that lower-class children, as a group, have lower IQs than middle-class children. However, when differences are found in the behavior of lower-class children and middle-class children, the IQ difference is but one of many factors considered in the interpretation of these differences. Workers look closely at their subjects' social milieux, the child rearing practices to which the children have been subjected, and the attitudes, motives, and goals which these children bring to the experimental situation. In contrast, when we deal with the mentally retarded, we often seem implicitly to assume that the cognitive deficiency from which our subjects suffer is such a pervasive determinant of their total functioning as to make them impervious to the effects of influences known to affect the behavior of the nonretarded.

This assumption can clearly be seen in a commonly employed research paradigm in empirical work with the retarded. Many studies, directed at illuminating differences in cognitive functioning between normal and retarded subjects, employ comparisons of institutionalized retarded children whose preinstitutional lives were frequently spent in the very lowest segment of the lowest socioeconomic class, with middle-class children residing at home. Such groups differ, not only in respect to the quality of their cognitive functioning as defined by the IQ, but they also differ greatly in respect to their total life histories and the nature of their current social-psychological interactions. When an individual of normal intellect is subjected to the social deprivation associated with institutionalization or is a member of a particular social class, behavior theorists are extremely sensitive as to how life experiences associated with such factors give rise to particular goals, values, attitudes, motives, and roles, and how such variables, in addition to formal cognitive ones, influence the individual's behavior. However, in the case of the retarded individual, we seem all too ready to believe that a cognitive deficiency makes one impervious to environmental events known to be central in the genesis of the personality of individuals of normal intellect.

In defense of workers who employ the paradigm noted above, it could be argued that one need not be very sensitive to motivational or personality differences between groups compared on tasks thought to be essentially cognitive in nature. In my opinion, such an argument is an erroneous one. Although it is unquestionably true that the effects of particular motivational and emotional factors will vary as a function of the particular task employed, the performance on no one task can be considered the inexorable product of cognitive functioning, totally uninfluenced by motivational and emotional factors. Evidence in support of this point can be found in numerous studies employing tasks thought to be essentially cognitive in nature, where differences in performance have been found to be associated with social class in IQ-matched individuals of normal intellect, and related to institutionalization in IQ-matched individuals of retarded intellect. All of this leads me to reject the often implicitly held view that the cognitive deficiencies of the retarded individual are so ubiquitous and massive in their effects that we may safely ignore personality variables on which our retarded subjects may also differ from those individuals of normal intellect with whom we compare them. This strikes me as little more than a reaffirmation of the following sound experimental dictum: You cannot safely attribute a difference in performance on a dependent variable to a known difference in subject characteristics (e.g., IQ), if the populations also differ on other factors which could reasonably affect, or have been demonstrated to affect, performance on the dependent measure.

The overly cognitive deterministic approach to the behavior of the retarded would appear to stem from more than the implicit or explicit assumptions criticized above. It is probably also the result of the relative absence of a sound and extensive body of empirical work dealing with personality factors in the behavior of the retarded. The dearth of such work has invariably been noted by scholars faced with the task of reviewing those efforts that have dealt with the personality functioning of the retarded (cf. Gardner, 1968; Heber, 1964). Had such a body of work developed over the years, it would have unquestionably played an important moderating role with respect to the overly cognitive deterministic approach that we have been discussing.

Not only has there been surprisingly little work done in the development and structure of the personality of retarded individuals, but many of the views advanced concerning the personality structure of the retarded have been surprisingly inadequate, in some instances, and patently ridiculous in others. In a recent paper (Zigler & Harter, 1969), Susan Harter and I pointed out how, in the early years of this century, the viewpoint became popular that individuals of retarded intellect were essentially immoral, degenerate, and depraved. As representative of this point of view, we quoted a 1912 statement made by one of our nation's pioneer figures in mental retardation, Walter Fernald:

> The social and economic burdens of uncomplicated feeblemindedness are only too well-known. The feebleminded are a parasitic, predatory class, never capable of self-support or of managing their own affairs. The great majority ultimately become public charges in some form. They cause unutterable sorrow at home and are a menace and danger to the community. Feebleminded women are almost invariably immoral and . . .

usually become carriers of venereal disease or give birth to children who are as defective as themselves .... Every feebleminded person, especially the high-grade imbecile, is a potential criminal, needing only the proper environment and opportunity for the development and expression of his criminal tendencies. (Reported in Davies, 1959)

Unfortunately, the intervening half-century has not witnessed a very great abatement in our cliché-ridden and stereotypic thinking on the personality of the retarded. A fairly recent book on mental retardation (Mautner, 1959) emphasized a number of unsavory personality traits from which the retarded appear to suffer inherently, including criminality and the lack of inhibitory controls. The persistence of the view that retarded individuals universally suffer from some particular character deficiency or personality trait was also recently pointed out by Gardner (1968) who quoted a number of current workers guilty of such stereotyped thinking concerning the personality of the retarded. Several thinkers (cf. Wolfensberger & Menolascino, 1968; Zigler, 1966c) have noted how this deficit approach to the retarded has been extended, in certain instances, to the view that the retarded represent some sort of subspecies or homogeneous group of less than human organisms.

One cannot help but wonder what factors in our thinking have perpetuated these overly simplistic and obviously erroneous views about the personality of the retarded. I believe that some of this error can be traced directly to a common, but not necessary, outcome of the taxonomic practice of categorizing and labeling. As mentioned earlier, men can be fairly easily differentiated with respect to the rate of their cognitive development and the ultimate level of cognition achieved. Consistent with the taxonomic activities which permeate much of the scientific endeavor, this ability to differentiate quickly lends itself to the categorizing and labeling of individuals along some dimension of intellectual adequacy. The grossest example of this is our typical textbook presentation of the distribution of intelligence, in which a line is arbitrarily drawn through the distribution so that it intersects the abscissa at the point representing an IQ of 70, with everyone below this point categorized as mentally retarded. If one is not careful, this straightforward and, certainly, defensible practice can subtly and deleteriously influence our general views concerning the essential nature of intellectually retarded individuals. If one fails to appreciate both the arbitrary nature of the 70 IQ cut-off point and the fact that we are dividing people on nothing more than the grossest overall measure of cognitive functioning, it is but a short step to the formulation that all those falling below this point compose a class of subnormals. Since the conceptual distance between "subnormal" and "abnormal," the latter with its age-old connotation of disease and defect, is minimal, the final easy step is to regard the retarded as a homogeneous group of organisms defective in all spheres of functioning and forever separated, by their very nature, from all persons possessing a higher IQ.

Again, clarity is in order. There is no question that retarded individuals differ from normal individuals in cognitive functioning. However, we must be on guard not to generalize from this and create a general difference orientation in our approach to the behavior of retarded and normal individuals. Unfortunately, just such a difference orientation appears to suffuse our thinking concerning the retarded. The bulk of our effort is directed at the discovery of how the retarded are different from the more intelligent members of our society, and very little attention is paid to how the retarded are similar to individuals of normal intellect. While the difference orientation may have a certain viability in the early stages of our investigation of cognitive differences between normal and retarded individuals, its value shrinks drastically when we are confronted with the issue of personality differences between the retarded and individuals of normal intellect. Indeed, the difference orientation in the personality sphere becomes totally indefensible when it generates some stereotyped view of personality functioning applicable to all retarded individuals. The great heterogeneity in personality functioning that we can grossly observe in a random sample of retarded individuals makes it rather unlikely that a particular setting on personality traits, e.g., dependency, hostility, anxiety, aspiration level, negativism, is an invariable or inherent consequence of intellectual retardation. Rather than attribute inherent personality characteristics to the retarded, it would be more parsimonious to view the development of the personality of the retarded as no different in nature than the development of personality in individuals of normal intellect.

Once one accepts such a view, he turns his attention away from personality traits thought to manifest themselves as an invariable consequence of intellectual retardation and toward those particular experiences in the socialization process which give rise to the relatively long-lasting, emotional and motivational factors which constitute the personality structure. Once a worker shifts his orientation in this way, he is quite ready to discover that the personality of a retarded individual will be like that of a normal individual in those instances where the two have had similar socialization histories. He would expect differences to the extent that the socialization of the two individuals' histories differ. Furthermore, he would not expect a personality pattern unique to retarded individuals and shared by everyone whose intellectual features led us to label them as retarded. Rather, he would expect variation in the personality functioning of a group of retarded to the extent that the group members have had different life experiences, just as he would expect such differences among individuals of normal intellect who have had differing experiential histories. Thus differences in personality functioning between groups of retarded and normal individuals, as well as intragroup variation in the personality functioning of both retarded and normal individuals, would be finally attributed to variations in socialization histories.

That some differences in personality functioning would exist between groups of institutionalized retarded children and noninstitutionalized middle-class children of normal intellect would be expected, not because all retarded children represent a universal personality type, but rather because institutionalized retarded children have had such depriving and atypical social histories.

Indeed, it is hardly surprising that certain groups of retardates differ from normals in personality functioning in light of these atypical social histories. However, again, we must remember that the specific atypical features of their socialization histories, and the extent to which they are atypical, may vary from one retarded child to the next. Two sets of parents who are themselves retarded may provide quite different socialization histories for their children. At one extreme, we may find a retarded child who is ultimately institutionalized, not because of lack of intelligence, but because his own home represents an especially poor environment. At the other extreme, a retarded set of parents may provide their children with a relatively normal home even though it might differ in certain important respects — values, goals, and attitudes — from the typical home in which the families are of average or superior intelligence. In the first example, the child not only experiences a quite different socialization history while still living with his parents, but also differs from the child in the second situation to the extent that institutionalization affects his personality structure (see Yarrow, 1964). Given the penchant of many investigators for comparing institutionalized retarded children with children of average intellect who live at home, the factor of institutionalization becomes an extremely important one. One cannot help but wonder how many differences discovered in such comparisons reflect the effects of institutionalization, the factors that led to the child's institutionalization, or some complex interaction between these factors and institutionalization, rather than some purely cognitive aspect of mental retardation.

To add even more complexity, the socialization histories of both institutionalized and noninstitutionalized familially retarded persons differ markedly from the history of those retarded individuals who are brain-damaged. The brain-damaged do not show the same gross differences from normals in the frequency of good vs. poor environments. In the face of such complexity, we need not consider the problem unassailable, nor need we assert that each retarded child is so unique that it is impossible for us to isolate the ontogenesis of those factors which we feel are important in influencing the retarded's level of functioning. Once we conceptualize the retarded as essentially rational human beings, responding to environmental events in much the same way as individuals of normal intellect, we can allow our knowledge of normal personality development to give direction to our efforts.

This does not mean that we ignore the importance of the lowered intelligence per se, since personality traits and behavior patterns do not develop in a vacuum. However, in some instances, the personality characteristics of the retarded will reflect environmental factors that have little or nothing to do with intellectual endowment. For example, many of the effects of institutionalization may be constant regardless of the person's intelligence level. In other instances, we must think in terms of an interaction; that is, given his lowered intellectual ability, a person will have certain experiences and develop certain behavior patterns differing from those of a person with greater intellectual endowment. An obvious example is the greater amount of failure which the retarded typically experience. But, again, what must be emphasized is that the behavior pattern developed by the retarded as a result of such a history of failure may not differ in kind or ontogenesis from that developed by individuals of normal intellect who, by some environmental circumstance, also experienced an inordinate amount of failure. By the same token, if the retarded can somehow be guaranteed a more typical history of success, we would expect their behavior to be more normal, independent of their intellectual level.

This last statement, alluding to the improvement of the behavior of the retarded through the manipulation of environmental events which affect their motivational structure, leads me to raise a note of caution. Rather knowledgeable workers in the area of mental retardation (Milgram, 1969; Zeaman, 1968) have attributed to me a motivational theory of mental retardation. This is an error. I have never asserted, nor am I now asserting, that the essential nature of the deficiency in retarded functioning is motivational. As I hope has been made clear in this presentation, as well as in numerous earlier ones, I consider the essential difference between retarded and normal individuals to be cognitive. Thus no amount of change in the motivational structure of the retarded individual will make him intellectually normal, when such normalcy is defined in terms of those formal cognitive processes discussed at the outset of this chapter. However, we can speak of improving the performance of the retarded on a task, through the manipulation of motivational factors, to the extent that variations in the performance of that task are influenced by motivational variables over and above the cognitive demands of the task.

This point becomes an especially crucial one when dealing with the everyday social competence of the retarded individual. No amount of change in his motivational structure will make it possible for him to become a nuclear physicist. However, rather circumscribed changes in his motivational structure may make the difference between successful and unsuccessful employment at an occupation whose cognitive demands fall within the limits of his cognitive ability. I have been impressed by the repeated demonstrations that the performance of many retarded on a variety of tasks is poorer than would be predicted from their general level of cognitive ability, typically defined by their MAs. It is my view that a great deal, if not all, of this MA deficit in performance is due to the attenuating effects of motivational factors. However, if these attenuating effects were removed and the individual functioned optimally in a manner commensurate with his general level of cognitive ability, he would still be intellectually retarded in terms of cognitive comparisons with same-aged individuals of normal intellect. Thus a concern with motivational factors in the performance of the retarded holds no promise of a dramatic cure for mental retardation when such retardation is defined in terms of its essential cognitive foundation. A motivational approach does hold promise of informing us how we might help the mentally retarded utilize their intellectual capacity optimally. Although not terribly dramatic, such a goal is not only realistic, but is of the utmost social importance in light of the now well-documented evidence that the everyday adjustment and/or competence of the bulk of the retarded residing in our society is more a function of the retarded individual's personality than it is of his cognitive ability. Such evidence bolsters a recurring theme in my thinking; namely, that as important as the formal cognitive processes are, their roles have been overestimated, especially with respect to those minimal daily demands of society which we consider when assessing individual social competence.

Over the years, then, my colleagues and I have attempted to delineate and, in certain instances, experimentally manipulate a number of motivational variables: variables not unique to the performance of the retarded, but ones particularly relevant to the behavior of the retarded, inasmuch as retarded children, as a group, tend to encounter certain events much more than do middle-class children of normal intellect. We have been interested in discovering the particular experiences which give rise to particular motives, attitudes, and styles of the retarded and how variation in these experiences leads to variation in the personality structure of individuals of both retarded and normal intellect. We have, in certain instances, been especially interested in demonstrating that the performance of the retarded, which has heretofore been attributed to his cognitive shortcomings, is actually the product of a particular motive. This interest does not mean that we have invariably championed the importance of motivational over cognitive variables, since it is clear that these two classes of variables can, independently and in interaction, both influence performance on any given task. It has only been through a fine-grained analysis of the performance on a variety of tasks by a number of groups of retarded and normal subjects with varying socialization histories that we have been able to attribute particular aspects of performance either to cognitive or motivational factors. We have also been aware that, while it is conceptually feasible to draw a distinction between cognitive and motivational factors with respect to certain behaviors, this division becomes extremely difficult if not totally artificial. However, in much of our work, each of these two factors has been sufficiently delineated for us to demonstrate how each, independently, may affect the child's performance.

Over the years, we have questioned several relatively orthodox views and have tried to divest ourselves of those preconceived notions which stand in the way of increasing our knowledge concerning the retarded child. While we have attempted to broaden our thinking concerning the retarded child, we have certainly not tried to replace older views with any new orthodoxy. Unfortunately, we are rather far from the construction of any very satisfying nomological network of interrelated personality constructs which will provide the ultimate explanatory system of the personality functioning of the retarded. Rather than having evolved any such theoretical edifice, we still find ourselves at the earliest stages of theory construction; namely, the sheer isolation and mapping of those personality variables and their genesis which we think are particularly germane to the personality functioning of various types of retarded children. Although not committed to any formal theoretical statement concerning personality, our group over the years has had a very strong commitment to a particular research strategy. Of utmost importance in our work is our continued attempt to remain sensitive to what our subjects themselves are doing and thinking when they are presented with experimental tasks. Workers in our laboratory are continuously cautioned to stay tuned in to the child and to avoid the researcher's egocentricity which often grows out of too strong a commitment to a particular theoretical view or system. It is this continuing sensitivity to the child which often has dictated the specific direction of our research. We have found that if one takes the trouble to observe children closely while they perform on experimental tasks, rather than being interested only in whether the child's measured behavior confirms or disconfirms some *a priori* hypothesis, the child's behavior will dictate either the study which should be pursued next or an entirely new area of investigation which must be entered. Given this overview of our thinking, as well as the research strategies which have directed our efforts, it would now appear appropriate to turn our attention to the research itself.

The Lewin-Kounin Formulation

Our work began a good number of years ago when Harold Stevenson and I became interested in the Lewin-Kounin rigidity formulation concerning the behavior of the retarded. (*see* Zigler, 1962a, for a complete discussion of this position and the controversy which has surrounded it.) So much of our earlier work stems from this position and the experimental findings that supported it that at least a brief overview of the Lewin-Kounin effort becomes essential. This important theoretical formulation has had considerable impact on our conceptualization of the retarded, as well as on the treatment and training practices devised over the years to help the retarded, and it continues to this day to engender much research in the area. This formulation states that, due to the very nature of the development of retarded individuals, they are inherently more rigid than are chronologically younger normal individuals who are at the same mental age level. This view derived initially from Lewin's general behavior theory. Within this theory, the individual is treated as a dynamic system, with differences among individuals derivable from differences in: (1) structure of the total system; (2) material and state of the system; or, (3) its meaningful content. The first two factors play the most important role in Lewin's theory of mental retardation. He viewed the retarded child as being cognitively less differentiated, i.e., having fewer regions in the cognitive structure than a normal child of the same CA. Thus, with respect to the number of cognitive regions, the retarded child resembles a normal younger child. However, in terms of the material and state of the system, Lewin (1936) argued that even though a retarded child corresponded to a normal younger child in degree of differentiation, they were not to be regarded as entirely similar. He explicitly stated that he conceived "the major dynamic difference between a feebleminded and a normal child of the same degree of differentiation to consist in a greater stiffness, a smaller capacity for dynamic rearrangement in the psychical systems of the former."

Lewin presented a considerable amount of observational and anecdotal material, as well as the findings of one experiment, to support his theoretical position. Unfortunately, Lewin's experimental findings were ambiguous at best. It remained for Kounin (1941a) to provide clear experimental support for the position that retarded individuals are more rigid than normal individuals having the same degree of differentiation, i.e., MA.

Kounin (1941a,b; 1948), building upon Lewin's work, advanced the view that rigidity is a positive, monotonic function of CA. It is imperative to note that by "rigidity" Kounin, like Lewin, was referring to "that property of a functional boundary which prevents communication between neighboring regions" and not to phenotypic rigid behaviors, as such. Thus, with increasing CA, the individual becomes more differentiated, i.e., has more cognitive regions, which results in a lower incidence of rigid behaviors, while, at the same time, the boundaries between regions become less and less permeable. Furthermore, while this lack of permeability in the boundaries between regions often results in behaviors which would be characterized as rigid, in some instances, it leads to behaviors which could be characterized as indicative of "flexibility." (For an example of this latter possibility, see the results of Kounin's lever-pressing task presented below.)

Kounin offered the findings of five experiments in which he employed older retarded individuals, younger retarded individuals, and normals. (It should be noted that the two retarded groups resided in an institution, whereas the normal children did not.) The degree-of-differentiation variable was controlled by equating the groups on MA. As predicted, the performance of the three groups differed on certain instruction initiated tasks, e.g., first being instructed to draw cats until satiated and then to draw bugs until satiated; and first being instructed to lower a lever and then to raise the lever in order to release marbles. As predicted from the Lewin-Kounin hypothesis, the normals showed the greatest amount of transfer effects from task to task, the younger retarded a lesser amount of transfer, and the older retarded the least amount of transfer. That is, following satiation on the first drawing task, both retarded groups drew longer on the second task than did normals, with the least cosatiation effects (longest drawing time on second task) being observed in the older retardates.

Kounin also found that the retarded subjects spent considerably more total time on the tedious drawing tasks than the normal subjects, a finding not derivable from the Lewin-Kounin formulation. This was attributed to the "rigid state" of the retarded which evidently spells itself out behaviorally in persistence on boring tasks. Another unpredicted and rather surprising finding was that the older retarded group had a negative cosatiation score; that is, they spent less time drawing on the first task than on subsequent drawing tasks involving highly similar figures. More will be said about this rather intriguing finding later.

On the lever-pressing task, the greatest number of errors, lowering rather than raising the lever on task two, was made by the normals, the least number by the older retarded, with the younger retarded falling between these two groups. One should note that on this task the lesser "rigidity," as defined by Lewin and Kounin, of the normals resulted in a higher incidence of behavioral responses often characterized as rigid, i.e., perseverative responses. One should further note that this lack of influence of one region on another in the performance of the retarded would be predicted only in those cases where the retarded individual is "psychologically" placed into a new region by instructions, e.g., "push down; now push up." In those instances where the individual must, on his own, move from one region to another, the Lewin-Kounin formulation would predict that such movement would be more difficult for the retarded than for the normal individual.

This prediction was confirmed by Kounin's concept-switching experiment in which the child was given a deck of cards which could be sorted on the basis of either one (form) or another (color) principle. In this experiment, the subject was asked to sort the cards and was then asked to sort the cards some other way. Here the normals evidenced the least difficulty, and the older retarded the most difficulty in shifting from one sorting principle to another, while the younger retarded again fell between these two groups. Thus, in the instance where a child is not psychologically placed in a new region but must move through a cognitive boundary on his own, it is the retarded who evidence the greater incidence of perseverative responses.

The Lewin-Kounin theory of rigidity in the retarded is a conceptually demanding one in that it sometimes predicts a higher, and sometimes a lower, incidence of "rigid" behaviors in retarded as compared to normal individuals. However, the fact that it generates specific predictions as to when one or the other state of affairs will obtain is a tribute to this theory. Kounin thus offered impressive experimental support for the view that, with MA held constant, the older and/or more retarded an individual is, the more will his behaviors be characterized by dynamic rigidity, i.e., less permeable boundaries between regions.

Stevenson and I (1957) conducted a study that was designed to test the validity of the Lewin-Kounin theory of rigidity. This study investigated the ability of normal and retarded subjects to acquire one response and then to switch to a new response in a discriminative learning situation. Moving from Kounin's postulate that the boundaries within the life space are more rigid in the retarded than in normals, Stevenson and I hypothesized, "that the solution of a reversal problem would require movement to a new region of the life space and that such movement would be more difficult for the feebleminded subject because of the more rigid boundaries separating the regions of the life space." As to the actual rigid behavior resulting from such rigidity in a reversal problem, Stevenson and I chose as our measure the incidence of previously correct responses during the solution of the second problem. It would appear that such a perseverative response following the switch is the most direct evidence that the subject has remained in a prior region and has not moved to a new region.

Three groups of subjects were used: an older retarded group, a younger retarded group, and a group of normal children, with the groups equated on MA. (As in the Kounin study, the two retarded groups were institutionalized and the normal children were not.) The results indicated a striking equivalence in performance among groups. They did not differ significantly on the number of trials required to learn the initial discrimination problem, the number of correct choices on the reversal problem, the number of subjects in each group who learned the reversal problem, or on the direct measure of rigidity employed, the frequency with which subjects of each group made the response on the reversal problem which had been correct for them on the initial discrimination problem.

Although the switching problem employed by Stevenson and myself was relatively difficult, the possibility still remained that this switching problem was too easy to allow differences between the groups to become manifest. In order to investigate this possibility, Stevenson and I conducted a second experiment, designed to investigate the performance of normal and retarded individuals on a more difficult reversal problem. On the basis of the findings of the first experiment, we rejected the Lewin-Kounin formulation, testing instead the hypothesis that rigidity is a general behavior mechanism. From this hypothesis, it may be deduced that the frequency with which rigid behaviors are shown is a function of the complexity of the problem. We predicted that the frequency of rigid responses (perseverations) would be greater for both the normal and retarded groups in the second experiment, utilizing a more difficult reversal problem than in the first experiment, but that there would be no differences between the groups. All predictions made for the second experiment were confirmed. These findings were in essential agreement with those of Plenderleith (1956) who also failed to find the type of differences in performance between the retarded and normals on discrimination learning and discrimination reversal tasks that would be predicted from the Lewin-Kounin formulation. The more recent findings with Balla (Balla & Zigler, 1964) were generally consistent with those reported in the Plenderleith (1956) and Stevenson and Zigler (1957) studies.

Social Deprivation and Motivation for Social Reinforcement

In an effort to evaluate the disagreement of our findings with those of Kounin, Stevenson and I directed our thinking to the differences in tasks employed across the two sets of experiments and, probably more important, the characteristics of the subjects, over and above their formal cognitive characteristics, which could have influenced their performance. In respect to the retarded groups, their most obvious characteristic was that they were residing in institutions. Thus we evolved the view that the performance of such subjects on tasks like those employed by Kounin could, at least in part, be ascribed to the social deprivation experienced by institutionalized subjects. Stevenson and I noted that, in our experiments, the subjects were required to learn two successive discriminations in which there was minimal interaction with the experimenter while, in Kounin's tasks, the response had been made primarily on the basis of instructions. Thus differences in rigid behaviors between normal and retarded individuals of the same MA in the instruction initiated tasks may be related to differences in the subjects' motivation to comply with instruction rather than to differences in cognitive rigidity. This hypothesis was based on the assumption that institutionalized retarded children tend to have been relatively deprived of adult contact and approval and, hence, have a higher motivation to procure such contact and approval than do normal children. At the time, this assumption appeared congruent with the view advanced by other investigators that both institutionalized retarded and institutionalized normal individuals exhibit an increased desire to interact with adult figures (Clark, 1933; Sarason, 1953; Skeels, Updegraff, Wellman, & Williams, 1938).

The first test of this motivational hypothesis was contained in a study by Hodgden, Stevenson, and myself (Zigler, Hodgden,& Stevenson, 1958). In an effort to employ tasks comparable to Kounin's instruction-initiated satiation task, we constructed three simple motor tasks, each having two parts and each allowing the experimenter to secure a satiation, cosatiation, and error score. The study deviated from Kounin's procedure in that two conditions of reinforcement were used. In one, the experimenter maintained a nonsupportive role and did not reinforce the subject's performance; in the second, the experimenter made positive comments and, in general, reinforced the subject's performance.

Two specific hypotheses were advanced: (1) Support has a reinforcing effect which results in an increment in performance over that found in nonsupport conditions; and (2) Interaction with an adult and adult approval provide a greater reinforcement for the responses of institutionalized retarded subjects than they do for those of normal subjects. Two retarded groups (a support and a nonsupport) equated on CA and two normal groups (support and nonsupport) equated on CA were employed. All four groups were equated on MA. Six predictions were derived from the two hypotheses. Five of the six predictions were fully or partially confirmed. It was found that:

1. Retarded subjects spent a significantly greater amount of time playing the games under the support than under the nonsupport condition, while normal subjects did not.

2. Retarded subjects spent more time on the games than the normal subjects in both reinforcement conditions.

3. There was a significantly greater difference in length of performance between support and nonsupport conditions for the retarded than for the normal subjects.

4. There was little difference in the cosatiation scores for normal subjects between support and nonsupport conditions. However, for retarded subjects, support not only resulted in lower cosatiation scores, but in scores that were negative in value (the subject plays longer on part two of the game than on part one).

5. Cosatiation effects were generally less for retarded than for normal subjects under both conditions of support and nonsupport.

6. The proportion of errors was not significantly different for normal than for retarded subjects.

In addition, a significantly greater number of retarded subjects stopped the games at points where the experimenter asked them if they wanted to play other games. This was interpreted as further indication of their greater compliance with instructions. (The error in this interpretation will be pointed out in a later section of this chapter dealing with the phenomenon of outer-directedness.)

The marked sensitivity of the retarded, as compared to the normals, to variations in the degree of social reinforcement, as well as the marked shift by the retarded from one social reinforcement condition to another in behavioral indices thought by Kounin to reflect cognitive rigidity, lent a certain amount of support to the social deprivation hypothesis. As pointed out earlier (Zigler, 1966c), this social deprivation interpretation of Kounin's findings is bolstered further by the fact that Kounin employed a procedure for selecting his retarded sample which led to the inclusion of only those retarded subjects who were highly motivated to interact with an adult. However, the findings of the study by Hodgden, Stevenson, and myself were not of the sort that would lead one to abandon totally the Lewin-Kounin inherent rigidity formulation. In fact, certain of our findings were reminiscent of those found by Kounin. Consistent with Kounin's results, we found that regardless of social reinforcement condition, our retarded subjects performed an inordinately long time on relatively boring and monotonous tasks. As Kounin surprisingly found with his older group of retarded, we found that our retarded subjects in the support condition played the second part of a two-part cosatiation task longer than they did the first part, even though both parts of the task were extremely similar. (I must confess that this strange increase-from-part-one-to-part-two phenomenon remained a mystery to me for several years. I think I began understanding this phenomenon, which will be discussed at some length in the next section, when I gave up trying to interpret it in terms of theories with which I was conversant and relied instead on a closer and more clinical observation of what the child was feeling, as well as doing, when performing such a two-part task.) In light of this, the Zigler, Hodgden, and Stevenson findings hardly constitute any death blow to the Lewin-Kounin rigidity formulation. At most, these findings indicate that the production of phenotypically rigid behaviors is also influenced by motivational effects, a view not very much at variance with Lewin and Kounin's own stance concerning motivational factors. At this point, what appeared to be in order was a more convincing test of the view that the Lewin-Kounin rigidity formulation lent little to our understanding of the grossly observable high incidence of rigid behaviors emitted by the retarded.

In what I hoped to be a more definitive test of our view that the rigid behaviors emitted by the retarded were a result of the social deprivation they had experienced rather than a product of any inherent cognitive rigidity, I did a study (Zigler, 1958, 1961) in which it was hypothesized that, within an institutionalized retarded population, a relationship should exist between the degree of deprivation experienced and the amount of rigidity manifested. The specific hypothesis tested was the following:

> The greater the amount of preinstitutional social deprivation experienced by the feebleminded child, the greater will be his motivation to interact with an adult, making such interaction and any adult approval or support

that accompanies it more reinforcing for his responses than for the responses of a feebleminded child who has experienced a lesser amount of social deprivation.

In order to examine the social deprivation experienced by retarded children, a measure that would reflect long-term deficits was required. Since the population of events which constitutes social deprivation has never been adequately delimited, the procedure employed in this study was to have raters evaluate the preinstitutional history of the child in terms of degree of social deprivation.

On the basis of these ratings, 60 retarded children were divided into two groups, high and low socially deprived. The groups did not differ significantly on either MA, CA, or length of institutionalization. The study employed a socially reinforced, instruction initiated, two-part satiation game similar to those used in earlier studies. Three of the four predictions derived from the hypothesis were confirmed. The more socially deprived subjects: (1) spent a greater amount of time on the game; (2) more frequently made the maximum number of responses allowed by the game; and (3) evidenced a greater increase in time spent on part two over that spent on part one of the game. The fourth prediction, that the more socially deprived subjects would make fewer errors, only reached a borderline level of significance. These findings would appear to call seriously into question the Lewin-Kounin rigidity formulation, since it is difficult to derive from this formulation an explanation of differences in rigid behaviors between groups of retarded children equated on both CA and MA. The findings offer further support for the view that the rigid behavior observed in retarded individuals is a product of higher motivation to maintain interaction with an adult and to secure approval from him through compliance and persistence. These results also offer evidence that the institutionalized retarded subjects' higher motivation to interact with an adult is related to the greater preinstitutional social deprivation such subjects have experienced. Furthermore, individual differences among the retarded in persistent and/or compliant behavior can be related to differences in the amount of social deprivation experienced. Since the persistence and compliance exhibited by retarded subjects have been found to be related to social deprivation, the prediction was generated, at that time, that these characteristics would also be shown by subjects of normal intelligence who have experienced similar social deprivation. (The fate of this hypothesis will be noted shortly.)

In discussing this last study, I am afraid that I have passed too lightly over what has remained a thorny issue in much of our work, namely, the nature and measurement of social deprivation. Once a worker turns his attention from the cognitive characteristics of the mentally retarded and focuses on the effects of social deprivation on the behavior of the retarded, he finds that he has entered a general arena of psychology which has an extremely murky conceptual foundation and is characterized by a rather vast literature, replete with inconsistent and contradictory findings. It will probably not surprise you if I state that there are few constructs in psychology that have been more frequently employed, yet more inadequately defined, than social deprivation. The definitional dilemma has been noted by Yarrow (1961), and has been aptly summarized by Gewirtz (1957) in his assertion that the concept of social deprivation has been loosely applied to certain events early in childhood which, in turn, are characterized as being antecedent to certain social behaviors. The problem, of course, is that there is little agreement as to either the early events or the subsequent behaviors.

In attempting to operationalize the social deprivation construct for use with institutionalized retarded children, I, initially, entertained the possibility of using length of institutionalization as a measure of social deprivation. Such a measure would meet the requirement of reflecting conditions operative through relatively long segments of time. In addition, this measure has whatever advantage lies in being perhaps the most widely used referrent of social deprivation. However, upon closer analysis, I came to the conclusion that institutionalization *qua* institutionalization is not a clear measure of social deprivation. There can be little doubt that the contemporary conditions of institutionalization must be a determinant of the child's current behavior. However, the results of such institutionalization are far from clear. A fact that has not been sufficiently recognized is that institutionalization is not, in itself, a psychological variable. At best, it refers to some vague social status of the individual. In order to relate institutionalization to social deprivation, one must designate specific social interactions in the institution that give rise to particular behavioral propensities. Given these qualms concerning institutionalization as a measure of social deprivation, another possibility came to mind: that perhaps the commonality in the positive findings of studies in which institutionalization was used as a social deprivation measure was due, not to common psychological features of institutions, but instead to the fact that most institutionalized children tend to come from homes which are relatively depriving. This possibility suggested that it was the preinstitutional social deprivation experienced by the retarded child that needed evaluation. (Within such a framework, institutionalization would be analyzed for its particular psychological features and for its effects viewed as interacting with the effects of the preinstitutional psychological environment. I will have more to say on this matter in the subsequent section on institutionalization.)

These considerations led us to the construction of a standard, objective measure of preinstitutional social deprivation. This instrument has been continuously refined over the years and a complete description of its current form is presented in a paper by Butterfield, Goff, and myself (Zigler, Butterfield, & Goff, 1966). Initial work on this scale began with the 60 children employed in the study just described. Two experienced psychologists were asked to read the social histories of these 60 consecutively admitted, familial retarded children and to independently rate each of them on a social deprivation scale. The scale consisted of nothing more than a line, evenly subdivided for reference into six areas: "very protected," "protected," "slightly protected," "slightly deprived," "deprived," and "very deprived." The possible range of scores was from 1 (extreme of "very protected") to 60 (extreme of "very deprived"). The judges were not instructed as to what constituted "deprivation" or "protection" beyond being told that the concepts were concerned with the amount and quality of the interaction that the child had had with important adults in his life. The judges were also asked to list for each child the specific factors in that child's social history which influenced their ratings.

At this early stage, there was considerable interest in whether the social deprivation construct was tangible enough to allow an adequate degree of inter-judge reliability. In spite of the vagueness of the concept, as well as the ambiguity of the instructions, the inter-rater reliability was found to be a respectable .77. This is especially impressive in light of the skimpy social histories with which the raters had to work and the attenuated range of the social deprivation scores. No less than 47 of the 60 children fell in the three deprived categories of the scale.

There is clearly some commonality in the early histories of retarded children to which experienced psychologists respond in deducing the amount of social deprivation experienced. In order to determine what these common factors might be, we turned our attention to the specific experiences of the child which the raters had listed as being important in determining their ratings. The most frequently listed factors and the frequency with which one or both judges noted them are presented in Table I. The data reported in Table I make it abundantly clear that the early childhood histories of the institutionalized familial retarded differ greatly from those children of normal intellect with whom the retarded are so frequently compared. Such grossly observable differences in the degree of early social deprivation experienced should act as a strong deterrent to those who insist on interpreting the inadequacies in the behavior of such retarded individuals solely in terms of their formal cognitive characteristics. (Some preliminary work [Zigler, 1962b] with our deprivation scale did indicate that the institutionalized organic retarded had experienced less preinstitutional social deprivation than did the institutionalized familial retarded.)

Using the items in Table I as a point of departure, social histories of a large number of retarded children in a number of state schools were examined in order to assemble a collection of gross items thought to be the experiential referents of social deprivation. Each of these items was then refined into a continuous variable and their reliability (inter-judge) and validity (relationship to performance on a social motivation task and to diagnosis, i.e., familial versus organic) assessed. This process continued over several years until the final form of the scale consisted only of items that could be clearly and reliably rated, even by raters who were untrained in psychology.

In addition to these items, the scale also includes a single subjective estimate of social deprivation which the rater assesses prior to scoring each of the objective items. The subjective scale has values from 0 (no deprivation) to 24 (severe deprivation), and was retained in order to capture nuances of deprivation which may not be reflected in the objective items. It was also felt that, with added use, the relationship discovered between the subjective rating and individual items would throw further light on the social deprivation construct and perhaps lead to its refinement. Our factor analytic work with this scale indicates that it yields four discernible components. These components are best viewed as reflecting the preinstitutional continuity of the child's residences, the attitude of his parents toward institutionalization, the intellectual and economic richness of his family, and the marital harmony of his family. In a recent study, Silverstein and Owens (1968) found a generally similar factor structure when employing the scale with another population of the institutionalized retarded.

This social deprivation scale with its four component scores was first used in a study by Balla, Butterfield, and myself (Zigler et al., 1968). This study had among its goals a further clarification of my earlier findings (Zigler, 1961) indicating a positive relationship between degree of preinstitutional social deprivation and motivation for social reinforcement as measured by how long the child would persist in playing a monotonous but socially reinforced game. By using the scale, we hoped to discover the particular aspects of preinstitutional social deprivation that resulted in the heightened motivation for social reinforcement. The Zigler, Balla, and Butterfield study was also directed at shoring up a weakness in my earlier investigation. At that time, the children I described earlier had already been institutionalized for an average of two years. This makes it difficult to attribute, unambiguously, the observed relationship between social motivation and preinstitutional social deprivation to preinstitutional deprivation alone. In the Zigler, Balla, and Butterfield study, all of the subjects were tested shortly after their admission to the institution (i.e., within three weeks). This study also differed from the earlier one in that the institutionalized retarded of both the familial and nonfamilial types were investigated.

The findings of this study provided further support for the general hypothesis that social deprivation results in a heightened motivation for social reinforcement. As in the earlier study (Zigler, 1961), a positive relationship was found between preinstitutional social deprivation and the effectiveness of social reinforcers dispensed by an adult. It should be noted that, in the more recent study, this relationship was found at the time of admission, whereas in

Table I

Frequency with Which One or Both Judges Noted Each of Seven
Specific Factors as Having Influenced Their Ratings

Factors in Social History	N
Child comes from an orphanage or has lived in several foster homes.	20
Child's parents are divorced or separated.	16
Child was abused (physical punishment, sex play) or neglected (inadequately fed or clothed) to the extent that legal action was taken to remove him from his home.	14
Child comes from original home in which he experienced considerable abuse or neglect, but no legal action taken to remove child from the home.	13
Mother or father institutionalized (mental hospital, institution for the retarded, or jail).	12
Child is illegitimate.	6
Mother verbalized her negative feelings toward the child	3

the earlier study, it was found at an average of two years following admission. The findings of this study go beyond the earlier ones by indicating that the deprivation-social reinforcement relationship holds for the nonfamilial as well as the familial retarded, and by implicating particular aspects of the preinstitutional history as critical, namely, the harmony and richness of the child's family and the attitude of his parents toward institutionalizing him.

Another test of the view that the incidence of rigid behaviors is a function of the greater social deprivation experienced by the institutionalized retarded child, rather than a function of his inherent rigidity, was carried out by Green and myself (1962). We employed three groups of subjects: institutionalized retarded, noninstitutionalized retarded, and normals. It was assumed that the noninstitutionalized retarded child has suffered less social deprivation than the institutionalized retarded child. All three groups were equated on MA, and the two retarded groups were also equated on CA. As in the earlier studies, only familial retarded children were employed. Again, a two-part satiation type task was used.

The Lewin-Kounin rigidity formulation would generate the prediction that the performance of the two retarded groups would be similar and that their performance would differ from that of the normal group. The social deprivation hypothesis would generate the prediction that the performance of the normals and the noninstitutionalized retarded would be similar and that their performance would differ from that of the institutionalized retarded. The latter hypothesis was supported, with no significant differences in performance found between the noninstitutionalized retarded and normals. Both of these groups differed significantly from the institutionalized retarded. Again, it was the institutionalized retarded who showed the relatively long satiation times, a perseverative behavior that has been employed as evidence for the inherent rigidity of the retarded.

We (Zigler, 1963a) conducted a further test of the view that perseveration on open-ended satiation type tasks is a result of an enhanced effectiveness of social reinforcers, stemming from the greater social deprivation experienced, rather than a product of an inherent cognitive rigidity. This study differed from the one conducted by Green and myself primarily in that it included a group of institutionalized normal children. In this study, institutionalized children of both normal and retarded intellect were found to play a socially reinforced satiation-type task longer than did groups of noninstitutionalized normals and retarded of the same MA. This greater effectiveness of social reinforcement for both institutionalized normal and retarded children as compared with noninstitutionalized normal and retarded children has also been found by Stevenson and Fahel (1961).

Crucial to the motivational interpretation of many of the studies discussed above is the view that the institutionalized retarded have been deprived of adult social reinforcement and are, therefore, highly motivated to obtain this particular class of reinforcers. Evidence offering further support for this view is contained in a recent study by Harter and myself (1968), in which we found that an adult experimenter was a more effective social reinforcer than a peer experimenter for the institutionalized retarded, but not for the noninstitutionalized retarded. Thus it would appear that the institutionalized retarded child's motivation to obtain social reinforcement is relatively specific to attention and praise dispensed by an adult, rather than a more generalized desire for reinforcement dispensed by any social agent, e.g., a peer. This differential effectiveness of peer and adult social reinforcement further argues against the view that the retarded are inherently rigid and will, therefore, perseverate on a dull monotonous task. Rather, how perseverative the retarded child is would appear to depend on the valence of the social reinforcers dispensed during the task. That peer reinforcement was not highly valued by the institutionalized child is not particularly surprising, in view of the general availability of this type of reinforcer in the institutional setting as has been found in an observational study by Balla (1967).

Balla's observational study constitutes an important missing link in the chain of evidence which we have been attempting to forge. Although there is a certain appeal to the assumptions we have been making, a crucial question remains: Do the social histories of the institutionalized retarded differ from those of noninstitutionalized children of normal intellect in the specific ways which we have been suggesting? If it is true that performance differences between normals and the institutionalized retarded are due to differences in experiential histories of adult social reinforcement, then these differences should be discernible at the level of gross observation. Balla conducted observations in the homes of noninstitutionalized normal and retarded children and in several institutions which housed children of both normal and retarded intellect. The findings of the Balla study provided direct observational support for the assumption of an adult social reinforcement deficit; with respect to the quantity and quality of adult social interactions, the institutionalized retarded were found to be much like the institutionalized normal groups, whereas the noninstitutionalized retarded were much like the noninstitutionalized normal groups. However, when the institutionalized retarded were compared with the noninstitutionalized normals, the comparison most often made in the mental retardation literature, the retarded children were found to interact with adults significantly less often than normal children. It is, therefore, not surprising to discover that when such institutionalized retarded children are placed in the situation where social interaction is readily available, they choose to remain in such situations longer than noninstitutionalized normal children who are more easily satiated on social reinforcers.

Although we have been couching this discussion in terms of the socially deprived child's heightened motivation for social reinforcement, it should be noted that such a heightened motivation for social reinforcement has itself been used as an indicator of an important phenomenon discussed in the general child development literature: namely, dependency. Thus, with an almost imperceptibly slight shift in terminology, we might conclude that the findings in this section indicate that a general consequence of social deprivation is overdependency. It would be impossible to place too much emphasis on the role of such overdependency in the institutionalized familial retarded and on the socialization histories that give rise to such overdependency. In a paper (Zigler & Harter, 1969) reviewing factors in the socialization of the mentally retarded, Harter and I concluded that, given some minimal intellectual level, the shift from dependency to independence is perhaps the single most important factor to enable the retarded to become self-sustaining members of our society. It appears that the institutionalized retarded must satisfy certain affectional needs before he can cope with problems in a manner characterized by individuals whose affectional needs have been relatively satiated. These affectional needs can best be viewed as ones which often interfere with certain problem-solving activities.

Evidence on this point comes from a recent study by Harter (1967), in which institutionalized retarded individuals took significantly longer to solve a concept formation problem in a social condition, where they were face-to-face with a warm supportive experimenter who praised their performance, than in a standard condition, where the experimenter was silent and out of view. The retarded subjects in the social condition appeared highly motivated to interact with an approving supportive adult, so much so that it seemed to compete with their attention to the learning task. Further evidence on this point may be found in Balla's observational study. When observing institutionalized retarded children in a schoolroom setting, he obtained evidence indicating that this type of child employs the school as a place to interact with adults in an effort to compensate for the lack of such interactions in the other segments of his life space. It thus appears that, just as in Harter's experimental situation, institutionalized retarded children in the school utilize this opportunity to satisfy their motivation for social interaction, rather than to learn.

Such findings suggest that because the severely deprived retarded are highly motivated to maximize interpersonal contact, they are relatively unconcerned with the specific solution to problems. Of course, the two goals will not always be incompatible, but in many instances they will be. Some evidence that this attenuating aspect of retarded behavior can be overcome has been presented by McKinney and Keele (1963) who found improvement in a variety of behaviors in even the severely mentally retarded following an experience of increased mothering.

Social Deprivation and the Negative Reaction Tendency

Although an atypically high motivation for social reinforcement appears to be an important factor in the performance of the institutionalized retarded, it can, by no stretch of the imagination, account for all of the reported behavioral differences in comparisons of retarded and normal individuals of the same MA. A recurring theme in our work has been the necessity for appreciating the complexity of the retarded individual. It has certainly not been our goal to replace the view that the retarded are to be understood in terms of their cognitive features alone, with the view that they are to be best understood in terms of some single motivational factor. The gross observation of the behavior of the retarded indicates that a wide spectrum of motivational factors are influencing them.

A phenomenon which appears to be at considerable variance with the retarded individual's increased desire for social reinforcement (a phenomenon I have sometimes labeled the "positive-reaction tendency") has been noted, namely, the retarded child's reluctance and wariness to interact with adults

(Hirsh, 1959; Sarason & Gladwin, 1958; Wellman, 1938; Woodward, 1960). This orientation toward adults (which I have labeled the "negative-reaction tendency") appears capable of explaining certain differences between the retarded and normals reported by Kounin, differences that have, heretofore, been attributed to the greater cognitive rigidity of retarded individuals. As noted earlier, Kounin employed a cosatiation-type task as one measure of rigidity. In this type of task, the subject is instructed to perform a response and is allowed to continue until he wishes to stop. He is then instructed to perform a highly similar response until again satiated. The cosatiation score is the measure of the degree to which performance on the first task influences performance on the second task. The theoretical positions of Lewin and Kounin, as well as Stevenson and Zigler, would predict that the absolute playing time of subjects on task two, after satiation on task one, would be greater than that of normal subjects. However, neither of these positions can explain the recurring finding (Kounin, 1941a; Zigler, 1958; Zigler et al., 1958) that, as a group, retarded subjects, under certain conditions, perform longer on task two than they do on task one. Groups of normal children, on the other hand, have invariably been found to perform longer on task one than on task two.

In an effort to explain the longer playing times of the retarded on task two relative to task one, I advanced the following hypothesis:

> Institutionalized feebleminded subjects begin task one with a positive-reaction tendency higher than that of normal subjects. This higher positive-reaction tendency is due to the higher motivation of feebleminded subjects to interact with an approving adult. At the same time, feeble-minded subjects begin task one with a negative-reaction tendency higher than that of normal subjects. This higher negative-reaction tendency is due to a wariness of adults which stems from the more frequent negative encounters that feebleminded subjects experience at the hands of adults. If task one is given under a support condition, the subject's negative-reaction tendency is reduced more during task one than is his positive-reaction tendency. (Zigler, 1958).

The institutionalized child learns during task one that the experimenter is not like other strange adults he has encountered who have initiated painful experiences (physical examinations, shots, etc.) with supportive comments. This reappraisal of the experimental situation results in a reduction of the negative-reaction tendency. When the deprived child is then switched to task two, he meets it with a positive-reaction tendency which has been reduced less than has been his negative tendency. The result, then, is that his performance on task two is lengthier than it was on task one. The finding that normal children exhibit a decrease in length of performance during task two, as compared to task one, follows if one assumes that they have a relatively low negative-reaction tendency when they begin task one. When normal subjects are switched to task two, it is the positive-reaction tendency which has been reduced more, through fatigue and satiation effects, than any negative-reaction tendency they might have had. The result, then, would be a briefer performance on task two than on task one.

Thus I suggested that the cosatiation score mirrors a particular set of motivational determinants, rather than inherent rigidity. This view was first tested in a study by Patricia Shallenberger and myself (1961). The cosatiation score was obtained on a two-part experimental task similar to those used in the earlier studies. The study differed from the earlier cosatiation studies in that three experimental games preceded the two-part criterion task. These experimental games were given under two conditions of reinforcement. In a positive reinforcement condition, all of the subject's responses met with success and he was further rewarded with verbal and nonverbal support from the experimenter. It was assumed that this reinforcement condition reduced the negative-reaction tendency which the subject brought to the experimental setting. In a negative reinforcement condition, all of the subject's responses met with failure, and the experimenter further negatively reinforced the subject by noting his lack of success. It was assumed that this reinforcement condition increased the negative-reaction tendency. (Ignoring the positive-reaction tendency was dictated by the assumption that this tendency was less open to experimental manipulation than was the negative tendency.) Two groups of retarded and two groups of normal subjects, all matched on MA, were employed. One normal and one retarded group were given the positive experimental condition, while the other two groups received the negative condition. All subjects performed on the criterion task under identical conditions, i.e., during both part one and part two all subjects received liberal amounts of verbal and nonverbal social reinforcement.

The most striking finding of this study was the confirmation of the prediction that both negatively reinforced groups would evidence a greater increase in time spent on part two over that spent on part one of the criterion task, than would the normal and retarded groups who played the experimental games under the positive reinforcement condition. This difference was such that the two groups receiving the negative condition played part two longer than part one, while the two groups receiving the positive condition played part one longer than part two. These findings indicate that cosatiation effects are not the product of inherent rigidity, but rather of the relative strength of certain motivational variables, i.e., positive- and negative-reaction tendencies. These tendencies and their relative strengths seem to be the product of particular environmental experiences and, apparently, are open to manipulation and modification. Thus the Shallenberger and Zigler study presents further evidence that differences in the performance on certain tasks of retarded and normal individuals of the same MA can be attributed most parsimoniously to different environmental histories and motivations.

The findings of this study did require us to broaden our views concerning motivational factors in the behavior of the retarded. Whereas the earlier studies emphasized the increased motivation to interact with and receive the support of an adult, the Shallenberger and Zigler study demonstrated the role of another motivational variable, the negative-reaction tendency. It would seem that the experiencing of that population of events, which has been described as socially depriving, gives rise to an increased desire to interact as well as a wariness of so doing. This conclusion gave further impetus to our concern with the discovery of those specific events which give rise to each of these opposing motivational factors.

Certain findings in the Zigler, Balla, and Butterfield study (1968) threw some light on the particular preinstitutional experiences of the child which give rise to the wariness and fearfulness of adults that we have labeled the negative-reaction tendency. These findings indicated that it was the marital harmony factor in our deprivation scale which was most related to the manifestation of the negative-reaction tendency. It is not terribly surprising to discover that the particular items in this factor include the nature of the marital relationships of the parents, the father's mental health, the mother's mental health, the father's general attitude toward the child, and the mother's general attitude toward the child.

The view that the genesis of the negative-reaction tendency was to be found in early socially depriving experiences, rather than in mental retardation per se, was central to a study conducted by Susan Harter and myself (1968). In this study, our two-part cosatiation task was once again employed to compare the negative-reaction tendencies of institutionalized retarded children with those of noninstitutionalized retarded children living at home with their parents, in homes that could be considered at least fairly adequate. In order to investigate just how general the child's wariness (i.e., the negative-reaction tendency) was, our subjects were further subdivided so that half of each group was socially reinforced by an adult and the other half by a child of normal intelligence. The institutionalized retarded were found to manifest a higher negative-reaction tendency than did the noninstitutionalized retarded. This greater wariness on the part of institutionalized as compared to the noninstitutionalized retarded was found in both the adult and peer reinforcement conditions. It thus appears that the institutionalized retarded suffer from a generalized wariness of strangers, regardless of whether the strangers are adults or children.

The cosatiation scores used to measure the negative-reaction tendency of the noninstitutionalized retarded were very similar to those found with normal children of the same MA. The finding that nondeprived retarded children are very much like normal children with respect to a general fearfulness runs counter to considerable anecdotal evidence. This led Harter and I to raise the possibility that the very simplicity of the task we employed may have obscured the noninstitutionalized child's fearfulness. Cromwell (1963) has emphasized the failure-avoiding nature of retarded children's performance, a phenomenon which also suggests a certain wariness or fearfulness. To the extent that such failure avoidance underlies the retarded child's frequently noted wariness, one would expect to encounter it primarily on complex or intellectually challenging tasks where failure is perceived by the child as a probable outcome. This explanation would not account for the performance of the institutionalized retarded children in the Harter-Zigler study, however. It may be, therefore, that the retarded child's wariness is best conceptualized as the product of two relatively independent factors: one involving those negative experiences with social agents which make him wary of other human beings, and the other relating to failure experiences on intellectual tasks, which cause him to be wary of tasks, rather than of people. If this formulation were true, one would expect the institutionalized retarded to be wary on all tasks presented by social agents, regardless of the task complexity. The noninstitutionalized retarded, on the other hand, should only be wary of tasks that are of an intellectually challenging nature.

Further evidence for the importance of the negative-reaction tendency in the behavior of socially deprived retarded children, be they institutionalized or not, is contained in the recent experimental investigation by Weaver (1966). He examined the negative-reaction tendencies of a group of noninstitutionalized retarded children obtained in a school district in a large urban area which had an extremely poor record of academic, social, and health adjustment. Among the tasks employed by Weaver was one developed in our laboratory which required the child to place a series of cut-out shapes on a long felt board, at one end of which sat an adult. In one experimental condition, the adult positively reinforced the behavior of the child, while in the other condition he made negative comments concerning the child's performance. Unlike the time measures used in earlier studies, Weaver employed a more direct measure of the child's approach and avoidance tendencies, namely, how far from the adult experimenter the child placed the shapes. Consistent with our thinking concerning the negative-reaction tendency, Weaver found that, over the series of trials, children in the positive reinforcement condition moved toward the experimenter, whereas children in the negative condition moved away from him. (The findings of a subsequent study [Klaber, Butterfield, & Gould, 1969] indicate that the two experimental measures used to date to assess positive- and negative-reaction tendencies, persistence in playing a dull but socially reinforced task, and how far from a stationary adult a child places himself are significantly correlated.)

Since positive- and negative-reaction tendencies, as we have been describing them, are hardly unique to children of limited intellect, we have pursued this line of investigation in a series of studies with children of normal intellect (Berkowitz, Butterfield, & Zigler, 1965; Berkowitz & Zigler, 1965; Irons & Zigler, 1969; McArthur & Zigler, 1969; McCoy & Zigler, 1965). These studies have all been directed at further validation of what has come to be known as the "valence position". Stated most simply, this position asserts that the effectiveness of an adult as a social reinforcing agent for a particular child depends upon the valence which that adult has for the child. This valence is determined by the relative amount of positive and negative experiences the child has encountered at the hands of the particular adult whose social reinforcer effectiveness is being assessed, and/or other adults in the child's past from whom he has generalized. The five studies noted above employed length of playing time on a boring satiation-type task as the measure of the adult's social reinforcer effectiveness. These studies have produced considerable evidence indicating that prior positive contacts between the child and the adult increase the adult's effectiveness as a reinforcer while negative contacts decrease it. If the experimentally manipulated negative encounters in these experiments are conceptualized as the experimental analogue of what the institutionalized retarded actually have experienced, then the often reported reluctance and wariness with which such children interact with adults becomes understandable.

It should be noted that further investigation of such positive- and negative-reaction tendencies, their interactions, and the specific events which give rise to them may clarify issues much more global in nature than the troublesome finding that, under certain conditions, retarded individuals will play a second part of a two-part cosatiation task longer than the first part. I specifically have in mind the current controversy over whether social deprivation leads to an increase in the desire for interaction or to apathy and withdrawal (Cox, 1953; Freud & Burlingham, 1948; Goldfarb, 1953; Irvine, 1952; Spitz & Wolf, 1946; Wittenborn & Myers, 1957).

In respect to retarded individuals, a logical conclusion here is that this wariness of adults and of the tasks that adults present leads to a general attenuation in the retarded child's social effectiveness. Failure of the institutionalized retarded on tasks presented by adults is, therefore, not to be attributed entirely to intellectual factors but must be interpreted in light of the atypically high negative-reaction tendency of many retarded individuals. This tendency motivates them toward behaviors, e.g., withdrawal, which reduce the quality of their performance to a level lower than that which one would expect on the basis of their intellectual capacity alone.

The Reinforcer Hierarchy

Another concept which my colleagues and I have advanced to explain differences in performance between normals and retarded of the same MA is that of the reinforcer hierarchy. This reinforcer hierarchy pertains to the ordering of reinforcers in the individual's motivation system from most to least effective. While the motivational factors noted previously can explain many of the normal-retarded differences found by Kounin, they cannot handle parsimoniously Kounin's finding that the retarded evidence greater difficulty than do normals on a concept-switching task. An early explanation of this finding, which I advanced (Zigler, 1958), relied heavily on the retarded child's heightened motivation to interact with an adult and the relationship of this motivation to the child's compliance. I suggested that, while this heightened motivation results in greater compliance when it increases the degree of social interaction, it may not lead to greater compliance when such compliance terminates the interaction as seems to be the case in Kounin's card-sorting task. Thus the argument can be made that the institutionalized retarded are thrown into a conflict between making a particular response which leads to the termination of the social interaction, and failing to make the correct response which results in the continuation of the interaction. Since normal children would experience this conflict to a much lesser degree, their performance would be superior on Kounin's concept-switching task.

I finally concluded that this argument, though plausible, could not satisfactorily explain Kounin's finding of a sizeable difference in concept-switching between normals and retarded. Furthermore, my argument contained an inherent weakness in the assumption that all of Kounin's subjects were aware that resorting the cards would result in a termination of the social interaction. A closer examination of Kounin's card-sorting task led me to deemphasize the importance of social interaction and focus instead on the relative weakness of the reinforcer employed by Kounin to motivate retarded children on this task. The only reinforcer obtained by Kounin's subjects for correctly switching concepts was whatever reinforcement inheres in being correct. Being correct is probably more reinforcing for the performance of normal than for retarded children, who may value the interaction with, and attention of, the experimenter much more than the satisfaction derived from performing the task correctly.

The hypothesis suggested here is that if equally effective reinforcers were dispensed to normals and retarded of the same MA for switching concepts, no difference in the ability to switch would be found. Such a hypothesis demands the assumption that the positions of various reinforcers in the reinforcer hierarchies of normal and retarded children differ. Basic to this assumption is the view that for every child there exists a reinforcer hierarchy, and the particular position of various reinforcers is determined by (1) the child's developmental level; (2) the frequency with which these reinforcers have been paired with other reinforcers; (3) the degree to which the child has been deprived of these reinforcers; and (4) a variety of other experiential factors.

Considerable evidence has now been presented either indicating or suggesting that the reinforcer hierarchies of middle-class children differ from those of lower-class children (Cameron & Storm, 1965; Davis, 1944; Douvan,

1956; Ericson, 1947; Terrell, Durkin, & Wiesley, 1959; Zigler & Kanzer, 1962). Emanating from this body of work is the view that middle-class children are more motivated to be correct for the sheer sake of correctness than are lower-class children. These studies attest to the feasibility of attributing the differences in performance between normal and retarded children on a concept-switching task to such differing reinforcer hierarchies, rather than to the greater cognitive rigidity of the retarded. Terrell *et al.* (1959) and Cameron and Storm (1965) found that middle-class children did better on a discrimination learning task when an intangible rather than a tangible reinforcer was employed, while lower-class children evidenced superior performance when the reinforcer was a tangible one. This social class finding is pertinent to the relatively poor performance of the institutionalized familial retarded on concept-switching tasks, since such individuals are drawn predominantly from the lowest segment of the lower socioeconomic class (Zigler, 1961). The importance of the specific reinforcer dispensed, in studies of the retarded, is further suggested by the Stevenson and Zigler findings (1957) that when tangible reinforcers were given, the institutionalized familial retarded were no more rigid than normal subjects of the same MA on a discrimination reversal learning task. Furthermore, on a concept-switching task identical to Kounin's (1941a), both retarded and upper-class children switched more readily in a tangible than in an intangible reinforcement condition. Contrary to Kounin's findings, no significant main effect associated with the normal-retarded dimension was found (Zigler & Unell, 1962).

This suggests that the differences obtained by Kounin (1941a) on his concept-switching task resulted from the comparison of retarded with middle-class children who valued the intangible reward of being correct much more than did the retarded. These studies further suggest that not only retarded, but lower-class children, in general, would be inferior to middle-class children when such a reinforcer is employed. However, middle-class children should not be superior to either retarded or lower-class children of the same MA when these latter children are rewarded with more optimal reinforcers, i.e., reinforcers high in their hierarchies.

This view was tested by deLabry and myself (Zigler & deLabry, 1962) in an experiment utilizing Kounin's concept-switching task under two reinforcement conditions with groups of institutionalized familial retarded, lower-class, and middle-class normal children. In one condition, Kounin's original reinforcer, the reinforcement that inheres in a correct response, was employed. In a second condition, the reinforcer was a tangible reward, a small toy. Half the subjects in each group received the tangible reinforcer and half received the intangible reinforcer for switching from one concept (either form or color) to the other. The reinforcement hypothesis and the predictions derived from it were supported by the findings. The retarded and normal lower-class children did better (fewer trials to switch in the tangible than in the intangible condition), while the normal middle-class children did slightly better in the intangible than in the tangible condition. Reminiscent of Kounin's results was the finding of significant differences among the three groups who received intangible reinforcers. However, no differences were found among the three groups who received tangible reinforcers. Furthermore, no differences were found among the three groups that exhibited maximal performance (retarded tangible, lower-class tangible, and middle-class intangible).

I (Zigler, 1963b) have argued at some length that shifts in the position of particular reinforcers in the individual's reinforcer hierarchy are related to changes in cognitive functioning associated with differing developmental stages. However, such factors do not appear to be the crucial ones when one discovers differences in the reinforcer hierarchies of normal and retarded children who have been matched on MA, and thus grossly on cognitive-developmental level. Such differences appear to be more appropriately attributable to the particular social learning histories of the children in question. For instance, in retarded populations, the incidence of failure is so high that training is often centered on doing one's best rather than being right. This deemphasis of right for right's sake alone would lower the motive to be correct in the child's motive hierarchy. Again, however, caution is in order. Although retarded children as a group may value being correct less than do middle-class children as a group, this may not hold for any particular child. The crucial factor is not membership in a particular social class or being retarded in intellect, but, rather, the particular social learning experienced by the child.

This point is aptly underlined in a recent study by Byck (1968), who examined the performance of institutionalized mongoloid and familial retarded subjects (matched on MA, CA, IQ, and length of institutionalization) on the concept-switching task employed both by Kounin and myself. Each group was subdivided, so that half of the children were reinforced for their performance with a tangible reward (a small toy), and the other half with social reinforcers, including the information that they were correct. A highly significant interaction was found indicating superior concept-switching for the mongoloids in the intangible as compared to the tangible condition, whereas the reverse pattern was found for the familials. This finding is consistent with the social class and reinforcer effectiveness literature noted above, if one remembers that institutionalized familials almost invariably come from a lower-class background, whereas the mongoloids are much more likely to come from the middle-class. It would appear that it is the social learning experiences acquired fairly early in the child's life and prior to institutionalization that are influential in determining the potency of particular reinforcers. Several investigators (Davis, 1941, 1943, 1944; Douvan, 1956; Ericson, 1947) have noted that the emphasis on being right is primarily a middle-class phenomenon and that this particular intangible reinforcer is more frequently paired with other primary and secondary reinforcers in middle-class than in lower-class populations. The enhanced effectiveness of tangible reinforcers for institutionalized retarded and lower-class children would appear to be due to the relative deprivation of tangible rewards, such as toys, experienced by these children.

Up to this point, our discussion of the reinforcer hierarchy has focused upon how particular reinforcers (e.g., a small toy or the verbal statement, "You're right") external to the child, but dispensed to him by some social agent, take on their effectiveness as a consequence of the child's general cognitive-developmental level and/or social learning experiences. In more recent work, we have shifted our attention to the more general phenomenon of the intrinsic reinforcement that inheres in being correct, regardless of whether or not an external agent dispenses a reinforcer for such correctness. This shift in our orientation owes much to White's (1959) formulation concerning the inherent and permeating nature of the effectance motive in man as a behavior system. Whether or not one accepts the view that the individual's need for effectance or mastery is a basic need that parallels certain other primary drives, there can be little question that White's effectance concept provides a rubric for a variety of behaviors that appear very central in the individual's behavioral repertoire from infancy through senility, e.g., the desire for optimal levels of sensory stimulation, manipulation, exploration, and curiosity. In a series of studies (Shultz & Zigler, 1970 Zigler, Levine, & Gould, 1966a,b, 1967) which we have conducted primarily with normal middle-class children from infancy through the elementary grades, we have obtained some support for the view that using one's cognitive resources to their utmost is intrinsically gratifying and thus motivating.

The adaptive features of such a motive for cognitive mastery are rather obvious; Child and I (Zigler & Child, 1969) have recently discussed the importance of such a motive in relation to the entire spectrum of socialization. Although it is my inclination to view the effectance motive as inherent and central to the human organism, I think that it differs from such primary drives as hunger and thirst. If these latter tissue needs are not met, the person dies. This is hardly the case with the need to be effective or, more specifically, to utilize one's cognitive resources to the fullest. To note that cognitive mastery is not life-preserving does not mean that it is automatically expelled from the arena of primary needs. One drive, widely accepted as a primary one, is sex, a drive whose satisfaction is also not life-preserving. However, it would be easy to conceptualize both sexual and effectance needs as life-fulfilling ones, when such fulfillment is defined in terms of the successful perpetuation and evolution of the species. A species would become immediately extinct if all procreation ceased. By somewhat the same token, the adaptive aspects of the effectance motive in the face of a continually changing environment plays an important role in the successful evolution of the species. Given this, it would not be surprising to find the human organism at the biological level programmed with such needs as sexual activity and cognitive mastery. However, such species programming does not guarantee that every member of the species will, at all times, be highly motivated by such self-fulfilling needs. Foregoing examples of more elevated sexual abstinence, one immediately thinks of the individual whose life experiences have been of such a sort as to lead them to be frigid or impotent. In terms of some hierarchy of motives, one could say that the sexual motive in such individuals has dropped from its normal place toward the top of such a hierarchy to some place near the bottom.

Analogously, one could conceptualize a situation in which cognitive mastery drops in the motive hierarchy as a result of experiences which either specifically extinguish this motive or as a result of the elevation and/or emphasis of other motives more important to physiological or psychological self-preservation. In the case of the retarded whose efforts after cognitive mastery so frequently meet with failure, such a motive could easily become associated with anxiety. As a result, the retarded individual would be more motivated to escape the painful anxiety associated with cognitive effort than he would to directly gratify the cognitive mastery motive. Such a process may underlie the considerable evidence that has now been presented indicating that retarded children are more motivated to avoid failure than to achieve success (Cromwell, 1963). (Other effects on the retarded of failure experiences will be discussed in detail in the next section.)

Susan Harter and I have been collaborating on a project directed toward operationally purifying the effectance motive construct and examining such motivation in groups of normal and retarded children. Initially, we attempted to construct and pretest a battery of tasks which we felt measured various aspects of this motivation to master, to explore, to conceptualize tasks as challenging problem-solving situations, to be curious, and to solve a task for the sake of being correct. Our original efforts were partially guided by our intuitive attempts to design a set of tasks which might reflect those behaviors which we have observed to be important in the development of the normal child, but seemingly absent or less predominant among the retarded populations we have tested in previous studies. These preliminary efforts resulted in a battery of five tasks, each measuring various facets of the behaviors noted above. We have now tested these tasks in a study involving three groups of subjects: normal children, noninstitutionalized retarded children, and institutionalized retarded children, all matched on MA. The evidence presented throughout this chapter led us to consider the institutionalized population of the retarded as differing from their noninstitutionalized counterparts on just those motivational variables which Harter and I were investigating.

The results of this study indicate significant differences among groups in the predicted directions on four of the five tasks. That is, the typical pattern which has emerged is that the normal children show the greatest desire to master a problem for the sake of mastery, to choose the most challenging task, to demonstrate the greatest curiosity and exploratory behavior; the noninstitutionalized children show less of this type of behavior, and the institutionalized children, in most cases, demonstrate the least mastery motivation. To date, we have looked only at these general group differences; however, currently we are looking at the relationships among tasks in order to assess the degree to which these tasks are intercorrelated and may represent components of some general motivational pattern.

Of some special importance, in the study just described, is not only that the retarded differ from normal children, but that groups of retarded children, matched on intellectual functioning, differ from one another in respect to a general motive which would influence a wide variety of behaviors. Again one finds support in this section for the view that many differences in the performance of normal and retarded children are a result of motivational differences which arise from diverse environmental histories and conditions.

Expectancy of Success

Another factor frequently noted as a determinant in the performance of the retarded is their high expectancy of failure. This failure expectancy has been viewed as an outgrowth of a lifetime characterized by frequent confrontations with tasks with which the retarded are intellectually ill-equipped to deal. That failure experiences and the failure expectancies to which they give rise affect a wide variety of behaviors in the intellectually normal has now been amply documented (Atkinson, 1958a, b; Katz, 1964; Rotter, 1954; Sarason, Davidson, Lighthall, Waite, & Ruebush, 1960). However, experimental work employing success-failure manipulations with the retarded is still somewhat inconsistent. The work of Cromwell and his students (reviewed in Cromwell, 1963) has certainly lent support to the general proposition that the retarded have a higher expectancy of failure than do normals. This results in a style of problem-solving for the retarded which causes them to be much more motivated to avoid failure than to achieve success. However, the inconsistent research findings suggest that this simple proposition is in need of some further refinement. One investigator (Gardner, 1957) found that retarded subjects performed better following success and poorer following failure compared to a normal control group. Heber (1957) found that the performances of normals and the retarded were equally enhanced following a failure condition, and that while success enhanced the performances of both normals and the retarded, the performance of the retarded was enhanced more than normals.

Kass and Stevenson (1961) found that success enhanced the performance of normals more than that of the retarded. Another study also found that failure had a general enhancing effect for both normals and the retarded, but that failure enhanced the performance of normals more than that of the retarded (Gardner, 1958). In a recent study by Earl Butterfield and myself (1965b), one factor capable of producing this type of inconsistency was isolated. We found that both normal and retarded children reacted differentially to success and failure experiences as a function of their responsivity to adults, i.e., their desire to gain an adult's support and approval. The nature of the difference between normals and the retarded in their reaction to success or failure experiences appeared to be determined by this latter variable. Among high responsive subjects, failure, opposed to success, attenuated the performance of retarded while improving the performance of normal subjects. Among low responsive subjects, failure, compared to success, attenuated the performance of normals while improving the performance of the retarded. (Again we see the error of conceptualizing either normal or retarded children as homogeneously reacting in some stereotyped manner to an environmental event.)

One problem involved in the success-failure experiments is that the experimental manipulations typically involved very simple, circumscribed experiences of success or failure. They do not constitute an adequate experimental analogue of the lengthy and repeated history of failure assumed for the retarded. In a study involving prolonged failure, a condition more representative of what the retarded actually experience, Zeaman and House (1960) found that their retarded subjects were unable to solve an extremely simple problem although they had previously been able to do so. As reported below, fairly clear results are also obtained when the experimenter simply assumes that the retarded have a "failure set," rather than attempting to see how such a set is influenced by one more failure or success experience.

Assuming that the inordinately high incidence of failure experienced by retarded children produces such a failure set, Stevenson and I (1958) tested the hypothesis that the retarded would be willing to settle for a lower degree of success than would normal children of the same MA. To test this hypothesis, we employed a three-choice discrimination task in which only one stimulus was partially reinforced, the other two stimuli yielding zero reinforcement. Although it is now clear that performance on such a task is influenced by a number of other factors (Gruen & Weir, 1964; Lewis, 1965, 1966; Stevenson & Weir, 1959, 1963; Weir, 1962, 1964), the Stevenson and Zigler rationale was that maximizing behavior (persistent choice of the partially reinforced stimulus) should be more characteristic of the retarded than the normal child since retarded children have come to expect and settle for lower degrees of success than have normal children. This rationale is consistent with Goodnow's (1955) analysis of the determinants of choice behavior. Goodnow suggested that greater maximizing behavior will be found when a subject will accept less than 100% success as an acceptable outcome, while less maximizing behavior will be found when a subject is expecting 100% success, or a level of success greater than that allowed in the situation. As we predicted, retarded children were found to maximize their choice of the partially reinforced stimulus to a greater degree than normal children.

Further support for the expectancy-of-success hypothesis was found in a second experiment (Stevenson & Zigler, 1958) in which normal children were given either a success or failure condition prior to performing on the partially reinforced three-choice learning task. It was hypothesized that a preliminary failure experience would lower the expectancy of success and thus lead to a higher incidence of maximizing behavior. As predicted, a higher incidence of maximizing behavior was found for children who had experienced prior failure than for children who had experienced success. We thus see again that if normal children receive the experimental analogue of the real life experiences of retarded children (in this instance, a low degree of reinforcement across a number of tasks preceding the criterion task), they behave in much the same manner as do the retarded.

It should be noted, however, that in the first Stevenson and Zigler experiment the obtained difference in maximizing behavior between the retarded and normals is consistent with a number of other positions. These findings are certainly consonant with the Lewin-Kounin rigidity formulation (Kounin, 1941a, b; Lewin, 1936). Within this framework, maximization (consistently responding to one stimulus) could be conceptualized as perseverative, stereotyped behavior, thus generating the prediction that the inherently more rigid retarded child would maximize more than the less rigid normal child of the same MA. Some support for this interpretation of the Stevenson-Zigler (1958) findings is contained in the work of Siegel and Foshee (1960) who found that retarded children were less variable in their response patterns than were normal children of the same MA.

A further test of the validity of our motivational explanation for the differences found in the performance of retarded and normals of the same MA on a partially reinforced three-choice problem was conducted by Gerald Gruen and myself (1968). A procedure for differentially testing the Stevenson-Zigler motivational and Lewin-Kounin inherent rigidity positions suggested itself. If it is the lowered expectancy of success stemming from a high incidence of failure experiences that causes the retarded to manifest maximizing behavior, then this same type of behavior should be found in children of normal intellect who have also experienced relatively high amounts of failure. Lower-class children would appear to have had such a background (cf. Gans, 1962). The motivational position would, therefore, predict similarity in performance by retarded and lower-class children on a partially reinforced three-choice problem. The position that rigidity is inversely related to IQ would lead us to expect a dissimilarity in the performance of these two groups and a similarity in the performance of lower- and middle-class children matched on IQs.

In the Gruen and Zigler study, groups of middle-class normal, lower-class normal, and noninstitutionalized familial retarded children of comparable MAs (approximately seven) performed on the partially reinforced three-choice learning task employed by Stevenson and Zigler (1958). In order to throw further light on the possible motivational dynamics influencing performance on this task, two experimental manipulations were also utilized. As in Stevenson and Zigler's (1958) second experiment (which employed only children of normal intellect), the degree of success experienced by children immediately prior to performance on the learning task was manipulated. One-third of the children in each group were administered a number of pretraining tasks in which they experienced a high degree of success; one-third were given pretraining tasks in which they experienced a very low level of success; and one-third did not receive any pretraining. The expectation here was that the low, as compared to the high, success condition would lower the child's general expectancy of success and thus result in more maximizing behavior on the learning task.

Penalty and no-penalty conditions were also included. Gruen and Weir (1964), employing the same three-choice probability learning task as Stevenson and Zigler (1958), found that penalizing children by having them give up a previously won reward for an incorrect response (defined as a trial on which the subject received no reward) resulted in greater maximizing behavior than did reward alone. In this study, in addition to examining the sheer number of correct responses made, the strategies employed by the children in attempting to solve a problem were also investigated. Earlier studies (Gruen & Weir, 1964; Stevenson & Weir, 1959; Weir, 1962) have demonstrated that, when confronted with this task, a common strategy of MA-seven children is a left, middle, right, or a right, middle, left response pattern, which accounts for about 50% of the total number of responses made. It was this specific pattern strategy which was investigated in the Gruen and Zigler study.

The analyses we conducted on the pattern of responding, i.e., the strategy of the child, provided a more fine-grained look at what the child was actually doing than that provided in the earlier Stevenson and Zigler study. The findings of the Gruen and Zigler study and the conclusions to which they led us were as follows: Across all trials, normal lower-class children showed the most maximizing (correct responses), and the least left, middle, right patterning of their responses, while the normal middle-class children showed the least maximizing and most patterning. Retarded children fell between these two groups on both measures. Penalty as opposed to no-penalty resulted in significantly more maximizing behavior and less patterning. No effects as a result of prior conditions of success and failure were found for the lower-class and retarded children. However, consistent with the findings of Stevenson and Zigler (1958), for middle-class children, the preliminary success condition resulted in less maximization (fewer correct responses) than did the other two conditions. Furthermore, while the preliminary success or failure conditions did not influence pattern response strategies of the lower-class or retarded children, they did influence those of the middle-class children. For this group, children who had experienced the preliminary failure showed the least amount of patterning while those who had experienced success evidenced the most patterning.

Examining performance across the 100 trials employed, the findings obtained on the correct-response measure, in conjunction with those obtained on the pattern-response measure, permit certain conclusions concerning the processes which mediate the performance of the three types of children. During the early trials, all children rely rather heavily on the pattern response, a strategy dictated by their cognitive level as defined by MA. Subsequently, the operation of a number of factors appears to determine the child's willingness to give up this cognitively congruent strategy for a maximization strategy which, although not meeting the goal of 100% success, does provide the best possible payoff. One such factor is the penalty involved in continuing to utilize the pattern strategy. Across all groups, the penalty condition (punishment) causes the child to give up the pattern response in favor of the maximization strategy. This shift to a different strategy in the strategy hierarchy would appear to be predictable from the Law of Effect. However, independent of penalty effects, the three groups continue to differ in their tendency to make patterns which, in turn, produces differences among the three groups in the number of maximization responses.

These remaining differences between the groups are not at all consistent with the position that the lower the IQ, the greater the rigidity. The findings do appear consistent with the expectancy-of-success hypothesis advanced initially. In the middle-class child, this expectancy is relatively high and, therefore, he is unwilling to settle for that degree of success provided by the maximization response. Given such a situation, he can do little more than continue with the patterning response which, at this MA level, would appear to represent a relatively complex strategy. On the other hand, the retarded and lower-class children have a lower expectancy of success and are, therefore, more willing to give up the patterning response in favor of the maximization response. The tendency for lower-class children to make fewer patterning and more maximizing responses is understandable if one remembers that the retarded children in this study were obtained from special classes, whereas the lower-class children were obtained from classes in which they probably had to compete continually with brighter children. While this factor may be offset by non-school experiences, it is very possible that the lower-class child in the middle-class oriented schoolroom has more failure experiences than the retarded in special classes conducted especially for them.

The importance of these success and failure experiences is suggested by the impact of the success-failure manipulations on the middle-class children in this study. As in the Stevenson and Zigler (1958) study, greater maximization was found following failure than following success. At the same time, success resulted in an increase, and failure led to a decrease, in pattern responding among middle-class children. It would appear that the preliminary success experience enhances the child's confidence in the pattern strategy dictated by his cognitive level, and thus increases his reluctance to give up this strategy when confronted with a problem which he thinks can be solved. This reasoning would appear to represent an extension of our expectancy-of-success hypothesis. The smaller number of correct responses on a probability learning task by a middle-class child would appear to be determined not only by the amount of success he is willing to settle for, but also by the amount of confidence the child has in his own cognitive strategy. That the retarded child has little confidence in his own cognitive resources will be pointed out in the next section of this chapter. It would not be surprising to discover that the low-class child, who typically experiences a high incidence of intellectual failure, also distrusts his own cognitive strategies and is, therefore, more willing to give them up than is the middle-class child.

This argument would have been strengthened had the success-failure effects found with the middle-class group also been found in the retarded and lower-class groups. However, as has been noted and demonstrated (Irons & Zigler, 1969; Zigler, 1964), it is naive to believe that simple short-term experimental manipulations of the sort used in this study would inexorably affect all children to the same degree. How these short-term operations influence behavior will ultimately depend on how they are mediated by the child. The findings of the Gruen and Zigler study suggest that, unlike the middle-class child, the retarded and the lower-class child have such entrenched attitudes and expectancies that short-term experimental manipulations of success and failure have relatively little effect on their performance. The fact that lower-class children of normal intellect are more similar in their performance to the retarded than to middle-class children of the same MA is consistent with other findings (Zigler & deLabry, 1962) and allows the conclusion that differences between the retarded and middle-class children on a probability-type task are due to motivational factors of the kind which have been discussed, rather than to any inherent cognitive rigidity of retarded individuals.

Reminiscent of certain findings of the Gruen and Zigler study are those of Odom (1967). Employing the expectancy-of-success hypothesis, this investigator also found that lower-class children were more willing to employ a maximization strategy on the task I have been describing than were the middle-class children. However, what must be emphasized is that it is not social class nor intellectual level, in and of themselves, which determine the child's expectancy of success and thus his performance on this particular learning task. Rather, it is the particular incidence of success or failure experienced by the individual child that determines his expectancy of success. Certainly, a very protected retarded child, who may not experience as much failure as one who is less protected, will thus have a higher expectancy of success. Analogously, not every child in the lower socioeconomic class has the same history of success and failure. Thus the performance of the child is more predictable when it is approached from a psychological point of view, rather than from a demographic, economic, or social class membership frame of reference.

This is exactly what was attempted in a recent study by Rae Jean Kier and myself (1969), which employed the same three-choice probability learning task used in the earlier studies. In this study, only lower-class and middle-class children of normal intellect were employed. However, two types of lower- and middle-class children were investigated. One subgroup of middle- and one subgroup of lower-class children were selected on the basis of their evaluation by their teachers as being successful in school. Consistent with the hypothesis advanced, we found that, independent of socioeconomic class, it was the children ranked as unsuccessful by their teachers who were the most willing to settle for a lower degree of success and thus adopt a maximization strategy on our partially reinforced discrimination learning task. The Kier and Zigler study also provided some, heretofore missing, direct evidence that performance on this task does indeed reflect the child's expectancy of success. Using a modification of a direct measure of expectancy of success, constructed by Diggory (1966), we found that performance on this measure was correlated with performance on our learning task. That is, those children with the lowest expectancy of success made more correct responses on our learning task (i.e., adopted a maximization strategy) than did children with a high expectancy of success. The findings reported in this section would appear to provide considerable support for the view that motivational factors determined by experiential events are important determinants in the child's problem-solving across social classes and intellectual levels.

Outer-directedness

Another line of investigation in our work has indicated that, in addition to a lowered expectancy of success, the high incidence of failure experienced by the retarded generates a style of problem-solving characterized by outer-directedness. That is, the retarded child comes to distrust his own solutions to problems and, therefore, seeks guides to action in the immediate environment. In an early study (Zigler et al., 1958), it was found that the institutionalized retarded tended to terminate their performance on experimental games following a suggestion from an adult experimenter that they might do so. Normal children tended to ignore such suggestions, stopping instead of their own volition. Originally, this finding was discussed in terms of social deprivation and heightened motivation for social reinforcement and was interpreted as reflecting a greater compliance on the part of the institutionalized retarded. The position here was that social deprivation resulted in an enhanced motivation for social reinforcers and, hence, greater compliance in an effort to obtain such reinforcement. (I think we see here a clear instance of how a commitment to a particular viewpoint leads one to avoid interpretations of data other than the ones to which he is committed.)

However, Green and I (1962) found that, while normal children again exhibited little tendency to do so, a higher percentage of the noninstitutionalized than the institutionalized retarded terminated their performance upon a cue from the experimenter. This finding is incongruent with the social deprivation interpretation, which would generate the prediction that the noninstitutionalized retarded would be similar to normal children in their sensitivity to adult cues. This dissimilarity in the performance of the noninstitutionalized retarded and normals led us to suggest that such sensitivity to external cues is most appropriately viewed as a general component of problem-solving, having its antecedents in the child's history of success or failure.

Of the three types of children which Green and I employed, the normal child would be expected to have had the highest incidence of success emanating from self-initiated solutions to problems. As a result, such a child would be the most willing to employ his own thought processes and the solutions they provide in problem-solving situations. Antithetically, the self-initiated solutions of the retarded would be expected to result in a high incidence of failure, thus making the retarded wary of the solutions provided by their own thought processes. This type of child should then evidence a greater sensitivity to external or environmental cues, particularly those provided by social agents, in the belief that these cues would be more reliable indicators than those provided by his own cognitive efforts. The retarded, in general, then, would be more sensitive to external cues than would normal children. The institutionalized retarded live in an environment adjusted to their intellectual shortcomings and should, therefore, experience less failure than the noninstitutionalized retarded. This latter type of child must continue to face the complexities and demands of an environment with which he is ill-equipped to deal and should, as we found, manifest the greatest sensitivity to external cues.

This general position was tested by Turnure and myself (1964). In a first experiment, we examined the imitation behavior of normal and retarded children of the same MA on two tasks. One task involved the imitation of an adult and the other, the imitation of a peer. Prior to the imitation tasks, the children played three games under either a success or a failure condition. The specific hypotheses tested were that retarded children would be generally more imitative than normals and that all children would be more imitative following failure experiences than following success experiences. These hypotheses were confirmed on both imitation tasks. To the extent that the behavior of normal children is considered the preferred mode, this study indicates that the outer-directedness of the retarded child results in behavior characterized by an oversensitivity to external models, with a resulting lack of spontaneity and creativity. However, it must be emphasized that heightened outer-directedness is not invariably detrimental to performance on problem-solving tasks.

Turnure and I conducted a second experiment (1964) in order to test further the hypothesis that retarded children are more outer-directed than normal children of the same MA. In this study, an effort was also made to demonstrate that outer-directedness may be either detrimental or beneficial, depending upon the nature of the situation. Normal children and noninstitutionalized retarded children of the same MA were instructed to assemble an item, reminiscent of the object-assembly items on the WISC, as quickly as they could. While the subject assembled the item, the adult experimenter put together a second object-assembly item. The hypothesis was that the outer-directedness of the retarded child would lead him to attend to what the experimenter was doing rather than concentrating on his own task, thus interfering with his performance. When the child had completed his puzzle, the experimenter took apart the puzzle that he himself had been working on. He then gave this second puzzle to the child and told him to put it together as quickly as he could. Here, the cues that the retarded child had picked up as a result of his outer-directedness should facilitate performance on the second puzzle. The predictions were again confirmed. The normal children were superior to the retarded on the first task, whereas the retarded were superior to the normal children on the second task. No statistically significant differences were found in the control condition in which the experimenter did not put together the second object-assembly task while the subject was working on the first. Further confirmation of the outer-directed hypothesis was obtained by a direct measure of the frequency with which the children actually glanced at the experimenter. As expected, the retarded subjects were found to glance at the experimenter significantly more often than did the normal children.

The findings of this study not only confirmed the hypothesis that retarded children are more outer-directed in their problem-solving, but also suggested the process by which the outer-directed style of the retarded is reinforced and perpetuated. There are undoubtedly many real life situations in which the child is rewarded for careful attentiveness to adults. However, it is also clear that there will be many situations in which such attending will be detrimental to the child's problem-solving. Across tasks, optimal problem-solving requires a child to utilize both external cues and his own cognitive resources. The retarded child's overreliance on external cues is understandable in view of his life history. The intermittent success accruing to the retarded child as a result of such a style, in combination with his generally lowered expectation of success across problem-solving situations, suggests the great utility which such outer-directedness would have for the retarded.

A further test of the hypothesis that retarded are more outer-directed than normals was conducted by Sanders, Butterfield, and myself (Sanders, Zigler, & Butterfield, 1968). The central question we addressed was whether the outer-directedness of the retarded, found on simple imitation and object-assembly tasks, also manifests itself in a standard discrimination-learning situation. The discovery that the retarded child's outer-directedness influences even his performance on a discrimination learning task would indicate that this style of problem-solving is a relatively pervasive one which should be taken into consideration in evaluating the general behavior of the retarded child. Groups of normal and retarded children of the same MA were compared on a size discrimination task that involved the presentation of an additional cue which the subject could use in making his choice of stimuli. Three conditions were employed: (a) one in which the subject's response to the cue would lead to success (positive condition); (b) one in which it would lead to failure (negative condition); and (c) one in which no cue was presented (control condition). The expectation was that the cue would be more enhancing in the positive and more debilitating in the negative to the performance of the retarded than for the normal children. Although some rather complex findings were obtained in the positive condition which lent some weight to the outer-directedness hypothesis, this hypothesis received its strongest support under the negative conditions. The retarded made significantly more errors than normals in the negative conditions. Furthermore, the retarded made significantly more cued than noncued errors, while there was no difference between cued and noncued errors for normals. Thus the retarded relied heavily upon the negative cue even though it led to errors, while the normals did not. This study thus provides further evidence of an outer-directed style of problem-solving in retarded individuals.

Further work on the outer-directedness hypothesis was conducted in a series of three experiments by Thomas Achenbach and myself (1968), in which this hypothesis was reformulated in terms of a distinction between two contrasting learning strategies, defined by the degree of reliance upon situational cues as guides to behavior. Achenbach and I described these two strategies as follows:

1. The cue-learning strategy was defined as problem-solving behavior characterized by a reliance on concrete situational cues, such that overt behavior is guided by the cues with little attempt being made to educe relations among problem elements.

2. The contrasting problem-learning strategy was defined as problem-solving behavior characterized by active attempts to educe abstract relations among problem elements in order to proceed from these relations to the solution of the problem.

This distinction is reminiscent of Tolman's (1948) distinction between "narrow strip" and "broad comprehensive" cognitive maps and Bruner's (1965) distinction between "extrinsic" and "intrinsic" problem-solving.

Although our procedure varied somewhat across the three experiments, essentially we utilized a three-choice size discrimination task in which a light came on in association with the correct stimulus. On the first few trials of this learning task, the light came on almost immediately. As the trials progressed, however, the interval between the onsets of the trial and of the light became longer and longer. Throughout the trials, the subject was occasionally prodded to make his choice of stimulus as quickly as possible. This procedure was intended to create a somewhat ambiguous situation in which the child could either continue waiting for the light to direct his choice, or begin responding to the abstract relation (relative size) among the problem elements. Correct responses before the light onset were utilized as the measure of the successful employment of the problem-learning strategy. Control groups were also employed in which groups of subjects learned the discrimination without any light cue present.

In our first experiment, we examined the performance of institutionalized retarded, noninstitutionalized retarded, and normals matched for MA. (As noted above, the noninstitutionalized retarded should be even more reliant on external cues than should the institutionalized retarded, because the environment of the latter, which is geared more to their abilities, reduces the failure experiences leading to reliance on external cues.) In the control condition, the learning performances of the three groups were quite comparable. As predicted, however, in the cue condition, the retarded relied on the cue significantly longer than the normals. Furthermore, the noninstitutionalized retarded relied on the cue significantly longer than the institutionalized retarded.

In a second experiment, groups of normals and noninstitutionalized retarded were presented the learning tasks immediately after experiencing either success or failure. In this experiment, some further control groups were established in order to allow us to assess whether waiting for the light cue inhibited learning of the size relation, or was just a conservative response strategy whereby the subject decided to wait for the light even though he knew that size determined which stimulus was correct. In this second experiment, we replicated the findings of our first experiment and also demonstrated that reliance on the cue by the retarded involved an inhibition of learning rather than caution in responding. Contrary to our expectations, our failure and success manipulations did not significantly influence the reliance on cues, either by the normal or by the retarded. However, during this study, we obtained some rather serendipitous support for our view that it is the relative incidence of success and failure experienced by the child that determines his outer-directedness as defined by reliance on cues. We discovered a class of 16 retarded children whose teacher employed teaching methods directed to the long-term manipulation of precisely those variables which we thought mediated outer-directedness. Observation of his classroom made it clear that he showered new pupils with success experiences and attempted to increase their self-esteem. Thereafter, he specifically reinforced what he called "figuring things out for yourself," rewarding independent thought more highly than correct responses. We examined the performance of these 16 retarded subjects on our learning task and we discovered not only that they relied on cues significantly less than our other retarded children, but that they relied on them less, albeit not significantly so, than did the children of normal intellect. Again, we see that it is not the retardation per se that produces the behavior, but rather the particular experiences to which retarded children are subjected.

In a third experiment, Achenbach and I (1968) found a significant correlation between imitation of an adult and the number of trials taken to give up reliance on the cue in the learning task by the retarded, but not by normals. This suggested that the reliance on external cues constituted a more general, less task-specific strategy for the retarded than for the normal child. However, the findings of a recent study by Achenbach (1969) indicated that, for normal children, the cue-learning strategy is not necessarily task-specific, since such cue dependency was found to be related to the normal child's impulsivity as well as to the higher intellectual processes involved in analogical reasoning. It thus appears that for normals and the retarded, reliance on cues in a discrimination learning problem is but one manifestation of a general style of problem-solving.

This general style of problem-solving, which we have been calling "outer-directedness," may be called into play to explain the great suggestibility so frequently attributed to the retarded child (e.g., Davies, 1959). Other studies by Hottel (1960) and Lucito (1959), which have demonstrated that duller pupils showed more frequent conformity to group decisions than did brighter subjects under ambiguous stimulus conditions where the group made the wrong decision, are in keeping with our views concerning outer-directedness. Lucito's interpretation of these findings was that, as a result of their previous experiences, the brighter children see themselves as successful in interpreting objective reality and as definers of social reality for others; however, the dull children have more frequently failed at interpreting objective reality and, therefore, have looked to others to define social reality for them.

Also consistent with other studies are our findings that it is the noninstitutionalized retarded child who must continually meet the expectancies of a world with which he is ill-equipped to deal, who is more outer-directed than the institutionalized retarded child who resides in a less demanding environment more geared to his intellectual shortcomings. Our findings are in keeping with those of Rosen, Diggory, and Werlinsky (1966), indicating that residential care is more likely to foster the retarded child's optimism and self-confidence than is the nonsheltered school in the community setting. These investigators found that, compared to the noninstitutionalized retarded, the institutionalized retarded set higher goals, predicted better performance for themselves, and actually performed at a higher level. Edgerton and Sabagh (1962) have also pointed out certain positive features of the sheltered institutional setting for the high-level retarded child. They note certain "aggrandizements" of the self which are available, such as the presence of inferior low-level retarded children with whom they can compare themselves favorably, their far greater social success within the institution, and mutual support for face-saving rationales concerning their presence there. This argument is similar to that presented by Johnson and Kirk (1950), who favor separate special classes for those retarded children in public schools, since they tend to be isolated and rejected in regular classes.

What must be emphasized at this point is that the retarded child is not more outer-directed than the normal child simply because he has a lower IQ. Within our present theoretical formulations concerning outer-directedness, how outer-directed any child will be would appear to depend on two factors: (1) level of cognition attained, e.g., mental age; and (2) the degree of success experienced through employing whatever cognitive resources he has available. Ignoring the second factor, it may be asserted that the lower the mental age, the more outer-directed the child, since such outer-directedness would be more conducive to successful problem-solving than dependency upon poorly developed cognitive abilities. With the growth and development of greater cognitive resources, the child should become more inner-directed, since such cognitive development reduces the child's dependence on external cues. Furthermore, independence training with increasing age is characterized by a continuous reduction in cues provided the child by adults which further reduces the effectiveness of an outer-directed style. Thus the shift from outer- to inner-directedness in normal development would be viewed as a product of both the increasing cognitive ability of the child and the withdrawal of those external cues which had previously made the outer-directed style an effective one.

This general developmental factor does not explain the findings discussed in this section, which indicate that the retarded are more outer-directed than normal children even when matched on MA. Apparently, in these studies, the crucial variable is not the level of cognition attained, but rather, the success or failure experienced by the child when employing his cognitive resources. It would appear that certain age expectancies are firmly built into our child training practices and that society reacts to a child more on the basis of chronological age than mental age. The normal child's mental age is commensurate with his chronological age, and he is continuously presented problems that are in keeping with his cognitive resources. With increasing maturity, he experiences more and more success in utilizing these resources in dealing with problems. The retarded child, on the other hand, is continuously confronted with problems appropriate to his chronological age but inappropriate to his mental age. These problems are too difficult for him and he does not experience that degree of success which would lead him to discard his outer-directedness in favor of reliance on his own cognitive abilities.

It may be hypothesized that outer-directedness, which is learned relatively early due to the rather effective cues provided by adults and peers, would generalize to a multiplicity of other external stimuli. This generalization would impel the child to attend to a wide variety of stimuli impinging upon him, since such behavior has been conducive to more successful problem-solving. Such a style should be given up relatively early in the development of the typical child, but should continue to be characteristic of the retarded child due to the inordinate amount of failure he experiences when relying on his own resources. One would probably describe a child who utilizes such a style as being distractible and, in fact, distractibility has often been attributed to the retarded child (Cruse, 1961; Goldstein & Seigel, 1961). The outer-directedness hypothesis suggests that distractibility, rather than being an inherent characteristic of the retarded, actually reflects a style of problem-solving emanating from the particular experiential histories of these children. Some support for such a view has recently been presented by Turnure (in press) who examined retarded children's glancing behavior and found that such glancing was motivated by information-seeking and was neither a type of random behavior which one would ascribe to a neurological problem, nor was it some vacuous orientation to salient social stimuli. Employing the view that distractibility reflects a particular type of problem-solving, one would expect this style of problem-solving and the trait of distractibility in normal children whose self-initiated solutions to problems have often been inadequate (e.g., the very young child), or the inappropriately reinforced child (e.g., the child whose parents make intellectual demands not in keeping with the child's cognitive ability).

Institutionalization

No discussion of motivational factors in the performance of the retarded would be complete without a consideration of the role of institutionalization. Understanding the effects of institutionalization on the behavior of the institutionalized retarded is not only important in its own right, but also plays a unique role in assessing a number of particular theoretical efforts concerning mental retardation. The reason for this is that many of the theoretical approaches presently being employed to explain the behavior of the retarded have been derived almost solely from the performance of institutionalized retarded individuals. I hope that I have made clear by now that it is a serious error to assume that the performance of the retarded reflects their intellectual retardation, uninfluenced by the effects of institutionalization. If one has any remaining doubts, I would refer him to those findings with the retarded which indicate that institutionalization is associated with a decrement in performance on a number of tasks thought to reflect important cognitive processes, including the quality of language behavior (Lyle, 1959; Schlanger, 1954), the level of abstraction on vocabulary tests (Badt, 1958), the ability to conceptualize an emotional continuum (Iscoe & McCann, 1965), discrimination learning (Denny, 1964), and ability to form a learning set (Harter, 1967; Kaufman, 1963). (Whether these deficiencies in the behavior of the institutionalized retarded reflect an actual change in intellectual capacity or are motivational in nature is, in my opinion, still an open question.)

Findings such as these, plus those emanating from the rather dramatic studies and reports of deleterious effects of institutionalization on the behavior of normal children, have made us all too ready to conceptualize institutionalization as some negative, monolithic effect which is constant across every individual who experiences it. Immediately contradicting such a negative view of institutionalization are the findings reported in the previous section that the protected environment of the institution results in the retarded child being less outer-directed, and thus more spontaneously utilizing his cognitive resources than is the case with his noninstitutionalized counterparts. Here again, however, caution is in order. Before one can assert that institutionalization will have some common effect, regardless of the particular institution in which the child finds himself, one must be prepared to argue that the particular social-psychological phenomena which mediate the effect are constant from institution to institution. It is difficult for me to see how such an argument can be defended when there has been so little systematic work done to discover the psychological features that are common to all institutions. I concur with Sarason and Gladwin (1958) in their amazement that so little programmatic work has been done in the investigation of the nature of institutionalization. I also find myself in complete agreement with the views of Cleland (1965) that we must go beyond a concern with such demographic characteristics as the size of institutions for the retarded and begin, instead, the painstaking search for the particular social-psychological characteristics and practices of institutions which might optimize the development of children who differ among themselves in respect to important psychological features.

In our work on institutionalization, we have, therefore, entertained two assumptions. The first is that institutions for the retarded differ among themselves in the effects they have on children who come to them for care. Our second assumption lends even further complexity to an already complex state of affairs. It has been our view that one and the same institution may affect children differently depending upon the child's personality dynamics, which may themselves have been determined during the preinstitutional history of the child.

A recent study by Earl Butterfield and myself (1965a) is illuminating with respect to how particular practices in institutions give rise to particular behaviors. In this study, we examined differences in children's motivation for social reinforcement in two equally large residential schools for the mentally retarded in the same state and with identical admission policies. The children in the two institutions were matched on a wide range of variables, thus allowing us to attribute any discoverable differences to the factor of the child's residence in one institution rather than the other. The social climates in the two schools impressed us as very different. We described the two institutions (A and B) as follows:

In institution A, every effort is made to provide a noninstitutional, i.e., homelike, environment. School classes, residential units at the younger age levels, and frequent social events are all coeducational. Meals are prepared in the living units, where the children eat in small groups. Emphasis is placed upon individual responsibility rather than upon external control by the staff. No buildings are locked and all children who are ambulatory move freely about the grounds to school, work, and recreational activities. Isolation is rarely used as a punishment. Essentially no security force is employed. There are many small residential units and a number of factors are considered before assigning a child to a unit, e.g., age, sex, intellectual level, the child's attitude toward the caretakers and other children residing in the unit, and their attitude toward him.

In institution B, little effort is made to provide a homelike environment for the children. School classes, all residential units, movies, and most other social events are segregated by sex. Meals are prepared and children eat in a large central dining room with virtually no individual supervision. Emphasis is upon external control of the children by the staff, rather than upon inculcating individual responsibility. All buildings are locked, and no child moves about the grounds unless attended by an employee. Isolation is frequently used as a punishment. A large staff of security officers patrols the grounds regularly. Residential units are all of the large, dormitory type, and no effort is made to group children except by the gross criteria of sex, age, and general intellectual level. The social climate at institution A strikes one as being much more conducive to constructive, supportive interactions between the children and their adult caretakers than the social climate at institution B.

In this study, we again employed, as a measure of how motivated a child was to obtain social reinforcers, his persistence on a monotonous task when such persistence was rewarded with either attention or attention plus verbal approval. As would be predicted from our earlier work on social deprivation and motivation for social reinforcement, we found that the children from the more unenlightened, depriving institution had a significantly higher motivation to obtain both types of reinforcement. Such differences between institutions in retarded children's responsivity to social reinforcement has also been found by Klaber *et al.* (1968), employing both persistence and interpersonal distance measures of the child's motivation for social reinforcement. In a recent study, Klaber and Butterfield (1968) postulated that rocking behavior in institutions was related to the quality of institutional care, and found not only differences in the incidence of rocking behavior between institutions, but also differences among wards within the same institution. In this same vein, Butterfield and I (Zigler & Butterfield, 1966) found institutional differences in the performance of the retarded on the concept-switching task employed by Kounin to assess cognitive rigidity.

Let us now turn our attention to the evidence concerning an interaction effect between the effects of institutionalization and the preinstitutional history of the child. Such an interaction was shown in a study conducted by Joanna Williams and myself (Zigler & Williams, 1963). After an interval of three years, we retested the children who still remained in the institution out of the original group of 60 children whose motivation for social reinforcement I had assessed previously (Zigler, 1961). Employing the same original measure of motivation for social reinforcement, we found that the motivation for such reinforcement had increased for the children who had remained. This is understandable if one assumes that institutional living is socially depriving and thus results in an enhanced desire for the attention and support of an interested adult. However, most striking in this study was the finding that the increase between the two testings in motivation for social reinforcers was related to the amount of preinstitutional deprivation experienced. Children coming from relatively good homes evidenced a much greater increase in their motivation for social reinforcers between the two testings than did children coming from more socially deprived homes. It thus appears that the general motivational effects of institutionalization depend on the preinstitutional history of the child, with such institutionalization being more socially depriving for children from relatively good homes, than for children from homes characterized by a considerable amount of social deprivation.

An unexpected finding of the Zigler and Williams study was that a general decrease in IQs of the children had occurred between the two testings. This change in IQ, discovered in the context of a study employing the amount of preinstitutional social deprivation as an independent variable, is reminiscent of a finding by Clarke and Clarke (1954). These investigators found that changes in the IQs of retarded children following institutionalization were related to their preinstitutional histories. They discovered that children coming from extremely poor homes showed an increase in IQ, with no such increase observed in children coming from relatively good homes. Zigler and Williams, however, found that the magnitude of the IQ change in their subjects was not significantly related to preinstitutional deprivation. Although this finding was inconsistent with that of Clarke and Clarke, it should be noted that the only subjects in the Zigler and Williams study who evidenced an increase in IQ were in the highly deprived group. The failure of Zigler and Williams to replicate the findings of Clarke and Clarke may be due to two factors: the subjects used by Clarke and Clarke were older and had been institutionalized at a later age than the retarded children employed by Zigler and Williams; and the IQ changes reported by Clarke and Clarke took place during the first two years of institutionalization, while the IQ changes reported in the Zigler and Williams study were based on five years of institutionalization. This latter factor becomes important in view of Jones and Carr-Saunders' (1927) finding that normal institutionalized children show an increase in IQ early in institutionalization, and then a decrease in IQ with longer institutionalization.

The work of Clarke and Clarke, Jones and Carr-Saunders, and others (e.g., Guertin, 1949) dealing with changes in IQ following institutionalization has given central importance to the intellectual stimulation provided by the institution, contrasted with that provided by the original home. This orientation suggests that the change is one in the actual intellectual potential of the person. The Zigler and Williams study suggests that the change in IQ reflects a change in the child's motivation for social interaction rather than an actual change in his intellectual potential. That is, as social deprivation resulting from increased length of institutionalization increases, the desire to interact with the adult experimenter increases. Thus, for the deprived child, the desire to be correct must compete in the testing situation with the desire to increase the amount of social interaction. That this conflict would be resolved in favor of the latter motivation is suggested by our work indicating that "being right" is relatively low in the reinforcer hierarchy of institutionalized retarded children. This argument would appear to provide the conceptual framework for Clarke and Clarke's finding that highly deprived subjects evidence an increase in IQ with relatively short institutionalization, while the less deprived subjects demonstrate no greater increase than a test-retest control group. One would further expect that, with increasing institutionalization, all children would exhibit a decrease in IQ, the phenomenon found by Jones and Carr-Saunders (1927), and one that appears in the Zigler and Williams study. Direct support for this view comes from the finding in the Zigler and Williams study of a positive relationship between the magnitude of the decrease in IQ and the child's motivation for social reinforcement, as measured by the amount of time the children performed on the satiation task.

It should be noted that the Jones and Carr-Saunders study involved institutionalized children of relatively average intellect, thus indicating that the dynamics under discussion here are the same for both normal and retarded children. Furthermore, the position advanced here is quite consistent with the findings for normal children obtained by Barrett and Koch (1930) and Krugman (1939); these investigators found that the greatest increase in IQ was obtained by children who showed the greatest improvement in their personality traits and/or by children who evidenced a marked change in the nature of their relationship with the examiner. Conversely, what must be emphasized with respect to lowered IQs is not the lowered test score, per se, but rather that the factors which attenuate these test scores will, in all probability, reduce the adequacy of many problem-solving behaviors performed in a social situation. More direct evidence indicating the effects of motivation and social factors on IQ test performance is contained in a recent study (Zigler & Butterfield, 1968) of IQ change in children attending nursery school programs for the culturally deprived. This study indicates that the typical IQ gain found among such nursery school children is due largely to the effects of those nursery school experiences which ameliorate debilitating motivational factors, rather than to any change in the child's formal cognitive structure.

Further light was thrown on these issues in a continuation of the longitudinal investigation of those children of the original 60 who still remained in the institution as long as eight years after my original testing (Zigler, Butterfield, & Capobianco, in press). These children were given our perseveration measure of motivation for social reinforcement five years and again, eight years after my original testing. (Thus 60 children were tested on this measure on an average of two years after initial institutionalization, and children remaining in the institution were retested three years, five years and eight years after the original testing.) As in the case of the three-year follow-up, in the later follow-ups we also examined changes in the children's IQs after added years of institutionalization. Unlike our three-year follow-up, in our five- and eight-year follow-ups, we found a generally decreased motivation for social reinforcement in the children. This is not terribly surprising since, by this time, the children were well into adolescence and should not be as motivated to receive praise on a very simple task involving little more than dropping marbles into a hole. It is actually reassuring to find such a general decrease in the population of the institutionalized retarded, since both normal and retarded noninstitutionalized children evidence a decrease in their motivation for social reinforcement (i.e., dependency) with added maturity (Lewis, Wall, & Aronfreed, 1963; Stevenson, 1961; Zigler, 1963a).

However, the most significant finding of the five- and eight-year follow-up was the discovery that the effects of preinstitutional deprivation interacted with the effects of institutionalization even after the children had been institutionalized this long. Children from highly deprived preinstitutional backgrounds showed a greater decrease in their motivation for social reinforcement than children from less depriving backgrounds. This finding is consistent with our three-year follow-up, and again indicates that institutionalization is much more socially depriving for children from relatively good homes than for children coming from homes characterized by a high degree of social deprivation.

These findings would appear to support my position (Zigler, 1966b) that social deprivation is a phenomenon that, once experienced, becomes built into the structure of the child and there mediates the child's interactions with his environment. Certainly, the effects of early social deprivation can be influenced by subsequent environmental events, but the effect of such subsequent environmental events do not appear to act upon the child in a mechanical manner. Rather, the effects of such conditions as institutionalization appear to be comprehensible only if viewed in terms of the child's mediational structure upon which such events are acting. This view, which emphasizes the long-term mediational role of early social deprivation, stands in opposition to the view that social deprivation effects are best conceptualized within a short-term model analogous to hunger (Gewirtz & Baer, 1958a,b). Within this approach, social deprivation effects are viewed as being easily built-in or reduced through the relative satiation-deprivation of social reinforcement.

In our five- and eight-year follow-ups (at which time the children had been institutionalized for seven and ten years, respectively), the interaction between the effects of preinstitutional social deprivation and institutionalization was also found in the change in IQ data. Following five years of institutionalization (three-year follow-up), the children showed a marked decrease in their IQs (Zigler & Williams, 1963). By the end of eight years, the drop in IQ had not only leveled off, but a number of children now showed an increase in IQ over that obtained at the time of their admission. As reported by Clarke and Clarke (1958), children showing such an increase were more likely to come from preinstitutional backgrounds characterized by a high degree of social deprivation. That a significant interaction between preinstitutional social deprivation and IQ-change consistent with that of Clarke and Clarke was found in the later follow-up, but not in the earlier one, is probably due to the fact that, by the time of the later follow-up, our children were more comparable in age to those employed by Clarke and Clarke.

The particular pattern of IQ changes, found across the years of our longitudinal study, lends credence to the view that IQ changes following institutionalization are due to motivational factors which affect IQ performance, rather than being due to changes in the level of primarily intellective factors. Further evidence that IQ changes following institutionalization reflect motivational dynamics, rather than changes in formal cognitive functioning, was provided in a recent study by Butterfield and myself (1970). In this investigation we employed our social deprivation scale to measure preinstitutional deprivation and examined the yearly IQs, beginning one year prior to institutionalization through five years of institutionalization, for groups of familial and nonfamilial retarded. In both groups, there was a general decrease in IQs following institutionalization. Although our results were somewhat complex, we did find that the magnitude of IQ decrease was related to the degree of preinstitutional deprivation among both types of retarded children.

That changes in both the child's motivation for social reinforcement and IQ following institutionalization are dependent upon the particular characteristics of the institution may be seen in the longitudinal component of the study conducted by Balla, Butterfield, and myself (Zigler et al., 1968). This study was originally discussed in the section on social deprivation and the child's motivation for social reinforcement. You will remember that in it we discovered that, at the time of institutionalization, a positive relationship was found between the children's preinstitutional deprivation and their motivation for social reinforcement as measured on our monotonous but socially reinforced task. The children, in this study, who had remained in this institution were retested on the same experimental measure three years later, and we also examined what had happened to their IQs over this three-year period. Although generally consistent with the motivational hypotheses which we have been advancing, the exact nature of the children's performance following three years of institutionalization in this particular institution was quite different from that reported in the three-, five-, and eight-year follow-up studies and the Butterfield and Zigler IQ-change studies discussed above, all of which were conducted in one and the same institution. In the three-year follow-up study (Zigler et al.),we found a significant decrease in the familial retarded children's motivation for social reinforcement. This finding disagrees with that of Zigler and Williams (1963) who found a significant increase in playing time following three added years of institutionalization. The most reasonable interpretation of this difference in findings is that the institution employed by Zigler et al. (1968) was not as socially depriving as the one used by Zigler and Williams. The fact of the matter is that the institution employed by Zigler et al. is generally considered to be one of the most enlightened in the country. It was the "good" institution in the study of motivation for social reinforcement (Butterfield & Zigler, 1965a). This study provided experimental evidence indicating that it is less depriving than another institution which impressed us as having a social climate more similar to that of the one used by Zigler and Williams.

However, in the Zigler *et al.* study, as in the Zigler and Williams study, there was a significant relationship between change in the children's motivation for social reinforcement following three added years of institutionalization and their preinstitutional history of social deprivation. Children with the better preinstitutional histories showed a smaller decrease in playing time between the two testings than did the children with the poorer histories. Thus it appears that, even in an enlightened institution, institutionalization is more socially depriving for children from less depriving backgrounds. This finding again highlights the error in conceptualizing institutional living as if it affected all children in the same manner. It would appear that living in this particular institution ameliorated the effects of preinstitutional deprivation which resulted in a reduction in the children's atypically high and probably debilitating need for social reinforcement. Again, it must be emphasized that this amelioration was more marked for children who experienced greater rather than lesser amounts of preinstitutional deprivation.

Some evidence was also found in this study that the child's wariness or negative-reaction tendency changed over the course of three years of institutionalization and that the magnitude of the change also interacted with the child's history of preinstitutional deprivation. Employing the time spent on each part of the two-part game measure of negative-reaction tendency discussed in a previous section, we found that the more deprived children were more wary at the time of admission and became less wary following three years of institutionalization, whereas the wariness of the less deprived children increased with institutionalization. Thus the interaction between preinstitutional deprivation and institutionalization on the wariness measure was in keeping with the interaction found for the motivation for social reinforcement measure.

In opposition to the Zigler and Williams finding of a significant decrease in IQ following a number of years of institutionalization, in the Zigler *et al.* study, the familial subjects were found to evidence a significant increase in IQs after three years of institutional living. This finding may be regarded as further evidence that the institution employed in this study is less depriving than the one used by Williams and myself. My colleagues and I have argued that changes in intelligence test performance of the sort found in this and the earlier study were due to changes in motivational factors which can influence the intelligence test score, rather than to changes in the subject's cognitive abilities.

Support for this view was also presented by Zigler and Williams in their finding that children who showed the greatest need for social reinforcement, upon retesting, evidenced the greatest decrease in their IQs. However, in the Zigler et al. study, no relationships were found between IQ changes and preinstitutional social deprivation, need for social reinforcement at the second testing, or changes in the need for social reinforcement between the two testings. Therefore, the Zigler et al. study, taken alone, offers little support for our motivational hypothesis that social deprivation results in an atypically high need for social reinforcement which, in turn, attenuates intelligence test performance. This hypothesis generates the prediction that IQ changes following institutionalization should co-vary with both the child's preinstitutional social deprivation history and his measured motivation for social reinforcement. Nevertheless, the pattern of findings across the Zigler et al. and the earlier Zigler and Williams study does provide some support for the motivational interpretation of IQ changes. In both studies, there were complementary changes in the need for social reinforcement and changes in IQ. In the earlier study, there was a marked increase in motivation for social reinforcement and a marked decrease in IQ. In the Zigler et al. study, a significant increase in IQ was found to accompany a sizeable decrease in the children's motivation for social reinforcement.

A complex picture thus emerges of the effects that the particular institution employed by Zigler et al. had on the behavior of the children investigated. Over the course of three years of institutional living, the children's motivation for social reinforcement and their wariness of adults underwent certain changes, with the magnitude and nature of these changes being influenced by the child's preinstitutional history of social deprivation. A comparison of the findings of this study with those of the earlier ones also indicates that different institutions for the retarded may have quite different effects on their residents. It thus appears that how an institution affects a child depends on both the nature of the institution and the life history of the child prior to his institutionalization. This view seems preferable to the more common one where institutions for the retarded are seen as equally depriving environments which exert uniform influences on all children.

In respect to IQ changes following institutionalization, it would appear that the retarded child's atypically high need for social reinforcement, as well as his wariness, compete with the production of correct responses in the testing situation and thus result in intelligence test performance lower than that dictated by the child's intellectual resources. To the extent that the child's need for social reinforcement and his wariness are ameliorated, one would expect an increase in IQ. A promising avenue for further research would appear to involve the isolation of particular motivational factors, such as the child's desire for social reinforcement, which may influence an IQ test score, and the investigation of the genesis of such factors in the preinstitutional and institutional experiences of the child. The importance of this work rests upon the fact that such motivationally induced changes in IQ performance would probably be found with respect to a variety of other performances typically utilized to gauge general social competence. Furthermore, such work would be of the utmost practical importance in light of the evidence noted earlier that motivational and emotional factors are more important than intellectual abilities in determining the institutionalized individual's prognosis for success in the community.

Personality Factors and the Everyday Adjustment of the Retarded

The research which I have now reviewed for you has been conducted within a framework which emphasized the systematic evaluation of the role of experiential, motivational, and personality factors. It is precisely an understanding of these factors, and their relationship to intelligence level, which will provide a better understanding of the socialization process in the retarded. For while the majority of the efforts and environmental manipulations designed to improve the quality of cognitive functioning in the retarded have been relatively unsuccessful (*see* reviews by Jones, 1954; Zigler, 1966a), there is a growing body of evidence indicating that certain motivational and personality factors relevant to social adjustment are considerably more modifiable. As Penrose (1963) noted, after a lifetime of work with the retarded:

> The most important work carried out in the field of training defectives is unspectacular. It is not highly technical but requires unlimited patience, goodwill and common sense. The reward is to be expected not so much in scholastic improvement of the patient as in his personal adjustment to social life. Occupations are found for patients of all grades so that they can take part as fully and usefully as possible in human affairs. This process, which has been termed socialization, contributes greatly to the happiness not only of the patients themselves, but also to those who are responsible for their care. (p. 282)

It is perhaps within this area of socialization that we can do a great deal to enhance the everyday effectiveness of the retarded. Both Burks (1939) and Leahy (1935) discovered that personality and character traits were more influenced by environment than was intellectual level. Such findings bolster the argument that there are many modifiable factors which are important in the determination of social adjustment. It is not rare to encounter individuals with the same intellectual make-up demonstrating quite disparate social adjustments. Perhaps, then, the important question concerning the socialization potential of retarded individuals centers less on the problem of how to improve their cognitive functioning than on the issue of how to maximize their adjustment, whatever their intellectual capacity may be.

Several reviews (Goldstein, 1964; Tizard, 1958; Windle, 1962; Zigler & Harter, 1969) of follow-up studies directed at assessing the adjustment of the vast majority of the retarded (IQs between approximately 50 and 75) have generated the same conclusion, namely, that there seems to be little relationship between cognitive status of these retarded individuals and their successful adjustment to the community. The soundness of such a conclusion is attested to most clearly in Windle's (1962) comprehensive review of over 100 studies dealing with the prognosis for the adjustment of the retarded discharged from institutions. The tendency to overemphasize the importance of intelligence in adjustment is made by his survey. Windle found that most institutions presume that intelligence is the critical factor in adjustment after release. He points out that the vast majority of studies on outcome "after release from institutions have reported no relation between intellectual level and later adjustment."

Windle goes on to state that there is some evidence (Grant, 1956; Krishef, 1957) which suggests a curvilinear relationship between outcome after discharge and IQ level, within the IQ range of 40 and 85. The tentative explanation for such findings is that, among the high IQ institutionalized retarded, there is a high incidence of personality problems which are more detrimental to extrainstitutional adjustment than is mild intellectual retardation in the absence of personality problems. Grant (1956), in examining the histories of his retarded subjects, found that the incidence of "character disorders," which he defined as persistent misconduct, was positively correlated with IQ. Tarjan and Benson (1953) have presented similar indirect evidence that the more intelligent subnormals released from the institution may have the most severe adjustment problems.

That personality factors are as important in the adjustment of the retarded individual as are intellective factors has been noted by numerous investigators (e.g., Davies, 1959; Penrose, 1963; Sarason, 1953; Tizard, 1953). In fact, many of the early workers in this country, such as Fernald and Potter, felt that the differences of social adequacy in that large group of borderline retarded was a matter of personality rather than intelligence. One of a number of studies which seem to confirm this view is a comprehensive survey by Weaver (1946) of the adjustment of 8000 retarded individuals inducted into the United States Army, most of whom had IQs below 75. Of the total group, 56% of the males and 62% of the females made a satisfactory adjustment to military life. The median IQs of the successful and unsuccessful groups were 72 and 68, respectively. Weaver's conclusion was that the "personality factors far overshadowed the factor of intelligence in the adjustment of the retarded to military service."

It has only been quite recently, however, that the specific personality factors relating to adjustment have been the object of more direct and systematic study. Shafter (1957), in attempting to ascertain those character-istics which best predicted successful adjustment of retarded individuals after release, first compiled a list of 66 variables which had been described in the literature and which he could objectify. He then compared the records of a group of 111 parolees who had been successful in adjusting to the community with a group of 94 who had been unsuccessful, i.e., had been returned to the institution. Included among those characteristics which contributed nothing toward predicting successful adjustment were IQ, age at discharge, length of institutionalization, and behavior record while an inmate. Among those 12 characteristics which significantly differentiated the successful from the unsuccessful parolees were truthfulness, obedience, attention to details and personal habits, (less) predisposition toward quarrelsomeness, and (less) display of aggressiveness in the institution.

The body of work on the social adjustment of noninstitutionalized groups also underscores the importance of personality factors. As Robinson and Robinson (1965) noted in their review of these studies:

> Success in obtaining and keeping a job is related to a large number of psychological and work-habit variables, including initiative, self-confidence, cooperation, cheerfulness, social mixing with other employees, respect for the supervisor, and understanding and efficiency in work. (p. 545)

Those factors which would seem to determine failure on the job have been studied by Collman and Newlyn (1956, 1957). They found that, among a group of retarded individuals who had been former special class pupils in England, those few who failed to keep their jobs were most often described by their employers as having some character deficiency, e.g., temperamental instability, inefficiency, and/or poor home conditions.

These findings, taken with the general literature on factors relating to the adjustment of the retarded, reveal that the characteristics associated with poor social adjustment include anxiety, jealousy, overdependency, poor self-evaluation, hostility, hyperactivity, emotionality, resistance, and failure to follow orders even when requests are well within the range of intellectual competence. To date, however, relatively little attention has been directed toward an examination of the processes through which such characteristics are developed in the maturing retarded child. Tizard (1958) makes a similar point in his review of the longitudinal and follow-up studies of the retarded, which he criticizes as being largely descriptive. He concludes with a plea that we "learn more about the basic psychological processes of the mentally subnormal, and the laws which govern their interaction and development." Similarly, Windle (1962) notes the narrowness of those studies which tend to focus on the total IQ score as the major prognostic indicator; he urges a more meaningful research approach in which a broader range of variables, e.g., personality factors, based on psychological theory, are examined.

While there is thus considerable agreement on the importance of personality factors, there has been too little attention given to the precise identification of these factors, their relative importance, and the socialization histories which give rise to such characteristics. The authors are certainly in agreement with the philosophy behind Davies' (1959) statement that, "The constructive efforts of (community) agencies are especially directed toward those elements of personality which have been shown not to be fixed, which are susceptible to improvement, and which are more decisive factors in socialization than intelligence alone (p. 216)." However, from his discussion of these rehabilitative efforts, it would seem that much of this work is being conducted on the basis of little established evidence. In the absence of such information, it appears that often, and perhaps necessarily, policy decisions are based on common sense, intuition, vague generalizations, and stereotypic beliefs about the retarded, e.g., the mentally retarded are "notably impressionable and easily influenced" (Davies, 1959).

Over the years, then, the research program I have reviewed for you has been directed at providing some hard evidence concerning the role of personality factors in the behavior of the retarded. We have tried to isolate the particular factors most relevant to the behavior of the retarded and have attempted to discover the particular experiences of the retarded which give rise to the particular characteristics of certain types of retarded children. While we have made some progress, certain notes of caution are in order. In my presentation, I dealt with one personality factor at a time. While this facilitated the presentation of the findings of a large number of studies, it may also have suggested that, when a retarded individual is confronted with a task, only one factor is operative. This, of course, is not the case. The psychological processes and the motive states, which we have been discussing, operate in combination more often than in isolation. This is merely to assert that the behavior of the retarded child on any task is a complex and multidetermined phenomenon.

It cannot be emphasized too strongly that much of the work reported in this paper is very recent. Many of the findings related to our hypotheses are more suggestive than definitive. However, it is my view that the factors we have been investigating are extremely important ones in determining the retarded individual's general level of functioning. An increase in our knowledge concerning these motivational and emotional factors, and their ontogenesis and possible manipulation, is mandatory before we can fully comprehend the behavior of retarded individuals.

References

Achenbach, T. Cue-learning, associative responding, and school performance in children. *Developmental Psychology*, 1969, 1, 717-25.

Achenbach, T. & Zigler, E. Cue-learning and problem-learning strategies in normal and retarded children. *Child Development*, 1968, 39, 827-48.

Atkinson, J. W. Motivational determinants of risk taking behavior. In J. W. Atkinson (Ed.), *Motives in fantasy, action, and society*. Princeton: Van Nostrand, 1958. Pp. 322-40. (a)

Atkinson, J. W. Towards experimental analysis of human motives in terms of motives, expectancies, and incentives. In J. W. Atkinson (Ed.), *Motives in fantasy, action, and society*. Princeton: Van Nostrand, 1958. Pp. 288-305. (b)

Badt, M. I. Levels of abstraction in vocabulary definitions of mentally retarded school children. *American Journal of Mental Deficiency*, 1958, 63, 241-46.

Balla, D. The verbal action of the environment on institutionalized and noninstitutionalized retardates and normal children of two social classes. Unpublished doctoral dissertation, Yale University, 1967.

Balla, D. & Zigler, E. Discrimination and switching learning in normal, familial retarded, and organic retarded children. *Journal of Abnormal and Social Psychology*, 1964, 69, 664-69.

Barrett, H. E. & Koch, H. L. The effect of nursery-school training upon the mental test performance of a group of orphanage children. *Journal of Genetic Psychology*, 1930, 37, 102-22.

Berkowitz, H., Butterfield, E. C., & Zigler, E. The effectiveness of social reinforcers on persistence and learning tasks following positive and negative social interactions. *Journal of Personality and Social Psychology*, 1965, 2, 706-14.

Berkowitz, H. & Zigler, E. Effects of preliminary positive and negative interactions and delay conditions on children's responsiveness to social reinforcement. *Journal of Personality and Social Psychology*, 1965, 2, 500-05.

Bruner, J. S. The growth of mind. *American Psychologist*, 1965, 20, 1007-17.

Burks, B. S. Review of M. Skodak, *Children in foster homes: A study of mental development*. *Journal of Educational Psychology*, 1939, 30, 548-55.

Butterfield, E. C. & Zigler, E. The effects of differing institutional climates on the effectiveness of social reinforcement in the mentally retarded. *American Journal of Mental Deficiency*, 1965, **70**, 48-56. (a)

Butterfield, E. C. & Zigler, E. The effects of success and failure on the discrimination learning of normal and retarded children. *Journal of Abnormal Psychology*, 1965, **70**, 25-31. (b)

Butterfield, E. C. & Zigler, E. Pre-institutional social deprivation and IQ changes among institutionalized retarded children. *Journal of Abnormal Psychology*, 1970, **75**, 83-89.

Byck, M. Cognitive differences among diagnostic groups of retardates. *American Journal of Mental Deficiency*, 1968, **73**, 97-101.

Cameron, A. & Storm, T. Achievement motivation in Canadian Indian middle and working-class children. *Psychological Reports*, 1965, **16**, 459-63.

Clark, L. P. *The nature and treatment of amentia.* Baltimore: Wood, 1933.

Clarke, A. D. B. & Clarke, A. M. Cognitive changes in the feebleminded. *British Journal of Psychology*, 1954, **45**, 197-99.

Clarke, A. M. Criteria and classification of mental deficiency. In A. M. Clarke & A. D. B. Clarke (Eds.), *Mental deficiency: The changing outlook.* New York: Free Press, 1958. Pp. 43-64.

Cleland, C. Evidence on the relationship between size and institutional effectiveness: A review and an analysis. *American Journal of Mental Deficiency*, 1965, **70**, 423-31.

Collman, R. D. & Newlyn, D. Employment success of educationally subnormal ex-pupils in England. *American Journal of Mental Deficiency*, 1956, **60**, 733-43.

Collman, R. D. & Newlyn, D. Employment success of mentally dull and intellectually normal ex-pupils in England. *American Journal of Mental Deficiency*, 1957, **61**, 484-90.

Cox, F. The origins of the dependency drive. *Australian Journal of Psychology*, 1953, **5**, 64-73.

Cromwell, R. L. A social learning approach to mental retardation. In N. R. Ellis (Ed.), *Handbook of mental deficiency.* New York: McGraw-Hill, 1963. Pp. 41-91.

Cruse, D. Effects of distractions upon the performance of brain-injured and familial retarded children. *American Journal of Mental Deficiency*, 1961, **66**, 86-92.

Davies, S. P. *The mentally retarded in society*. New York: Columbia University Press, 1959.

Davis, A. American status systems and the socialization of the child. *American Sociological Review*, 1941, **6**, 234-54.

Davis, A. Child training and social class. In R. Barker, J. Kounin, & M. Wright (Eds.), *Child behavior and development*. New York: McGraw-Hill, 1943. Pp. 607-19.

Davis, A. Socialization and adolescent personality. In *Adolescence. National society for the study of education*, Part I. Chicago: National Society for the Study of Education, 1944. Pp. 198-216.

Denny, M. R. Research in learning and performance. In H. A. Stevens & R. Heber (Eds.), *Mental retardation: A review of research*. Chicago: University of Chicago Press, 1964. Pp. 100-36.

Diggory, J. C. *Self-evaluation: Concepts and studies*. New York: Wiley, 1966.

Douvan, E. Social status and success striving. *Journal of Abnormal and Social Psychology*, 1956, **52**, 219-23.

Edgerton, R. B. & Sabagh, G. From mortification to aggrandizement: Changing self-conception in the careers of the mentally retarded. *Psychiatry*, 1962, **25**, 263-72.

Ericson, M. Social status and child rearing practices. In T. M. Newcomb & E. L. Hartley (Eds.), *Readings in social psychology*. New York: Holt, Rinehart & Winston, 1947.

Freud, A. & Burlingham, D. *Infants without families*. New York: International Universities Press, 1948.

Gans, H. J. *The urban villagers*. New York: Free Press, 1962.

Gardner, W. I. Effects of interpolated success and failure on motor task performance in mental defectives. Paper read at Southeastern Psychological Association, Nashville, 1957.

Gardner, W. I. Reactions of intellectually normal and retarded boys after experimentally induced failure: A social learning theory interpretation. Unpublished doctoral dissertation, George Peabody College for Teachers, 1958.

Gardner, W. I. Personality characteristics of the mentally retarded: Review and critique. In H. J. Prehm, L. A. Hamerlynck, & J. E. Crosson (Eds.), *Behavioral Research in Mental Retardation*, Rehabilitation Research and Training Center in Mental Retardation. Eugene, Ore.: University of Oregon Press, 1968. No. 1. Pp. 53-68.

Gewirtz, J. Social deprivation and dependency: A learning analysis. Paper presented at American Psychological Association meeting, New York City, 1957.

Gewirtz, J. & Baer, D. M. Deprivation and satiation of social reinforcers as drive conditions. *Journal of Abnormal and Social Psychology*, 1958, **57**, 165-72. (a)

Gewirtz, J. & Baer, D. M. The effects of brief social deprivation on behaviors for a social reinforcer. *Journal of Abnormal and Social Psychology*, 1958, **56**, 49-56. (b)

Goldfarb, W. The effects of early institutional care on adolescent personality. *Journal of Experimental Education*, 1953, **12**, 106-29.

Goldstein, H. Social and occupation adjustment. In H. A. Stevens & R. Heber (Eds.), *Mental retardation*. Chicago: University of Chicago Press, 1964. Pp. 214-58.

Goldstein, H. & Seigle, D. Characteristics of educable mentally handicapped children. In W. Rothstein (Ed.), *Mental retardation: Readings and resources*. New York: Holt, Rinehart & Winston, 1961.

Goldstein, K. Concerning rigidity. *Character and Personality*, 1942-43, **11**, 209-26.

Goodnow, J. J. Determinants of choice distribution in two-choice situations. *American Journal of Psychology*, 1955, **68**, 106-16.

Grant, J. R. Results of institutional treatment of juvenile mental defectives over a 30-year period. *Canadian Medical Association Journal*, 1956, **75**, 918-21.

Green, C. & Zigler, E. Social deprivation and the performance of feeble-minded and normal children on a satiation type task. *Child Development*, 1962, **33**, 499-508.

Gruen, G. E. & Weir, M. W. Effect of instructions, penalty, and age on probability learning. *Child Development*, 1964, **35**, 265-73.

Gruen, G. E. & Zigler, E. Expectancy of success and the probability learning of middle-class, lower-class, and retarded children. *Journal of Abnormal Psychology*, 1968, **73**, 343-52.

Guertin, W. H. Mental growth in pseudo-feeblemindedness. *Journal of Clinical Psychology*, 1949, **5**, 414-18.

Harter, S. Mental age, IQ, and motivational factors in the discrimination learning set performance of normal and retarded children. *Journal of Experimental Child Psychology*, 1967, **5**, 123-41.

Harter, S. & Zigler, E. Effectiveness of adult and peer reinforcement on the performance of institutionalized and noninstitutionalized retardates. *Journal of Abnormal Psychology*, 1968, **73**, 144-49.

Heber, R. F. Expectancy and expectancy changes in normal and mentally retarded boys. Unpublished doctoral dissertation, George Peabody College for Teachers, 1957.

Heber, R. F. Personality. In H. A. Stevens & R. Heber (Eds.), *Mental retardation: A review of research*. Chicago: University of Chicago Press, 1964. Pp. 143-74.

Hirsh, E. A. The adaptive significance of commonly described behavior of the mentally retarded. *American Journal of Mental Deficiency*, 1959, **63**, 639-46.

Hottel, J. V. The influence of age and intelligence on independence-conformity behavior of children. Unpublished doctoral dissertation, George Peabody College for Teachers, 1960.

Inhelder, B. *The diagnosis of reasoning in the mentally retarded*. New York: John Day, 1968.

Irons, N. & Zigler, E. Children's responsiveness to social reinforcement as a function of short term preliminary social interactions and long-term social deprivation. *Developmental Psychology*, 1969, **1**, 402-09.

Irvine, E. Observations on the aims and methods of child rearing in communal settlements in Israel. *Human Relations*, 1952, **5**, 247-75.

Iscoe, I. & McCann, B. The perception of an emotional continuum by older and younger mental retardates. *Journal of Personality and Social Psychology*, 1965, **1**, 383-85.

Johnson, G. O. & Kirk, S. A. Are mentally handicapped children segregated in the regular grades? *Exceptional Children*, 1950, **17**, 65-68.

Jones, D. & Carr-Saunders, A. The relation between intelligence and social status among orphan children. *British Journal of Psychology*, 1927, **17**, 343-64.

Jones, H. E. The environment and mental development. In L. Carmichael (Ed.), *Manual of child psychology*. (2nd ed.) New York: Wiley, 1954. Pp. 631-96.

Kass, N. & Stevenson, H. W. The effect of pretraining reinforcement conditions on learning by normal and retarded children. *American Journal of Mental Deficiency*, 1961, **66**, 76-80.

Katz, I. Review of evidence relating to effects of desegregation on the intellectual performance of Negroes. *American Psychologist*, 1964, **19**, 381-99.

Kaufman, M. The formation of a learning set in institutionalized and noninstitutionalized mental defectives. *American Journal of Mental Deficiency*, 1963, **67**, 601-05.

Kier, R. J. & Zigler, E. Probability learning strategies of lower- and middle-class children and the expectancy of success hypothesis. Unpublished manuscript, Yale University, 1969.

Klaber, M. M. & Butterfield, E. C. Stereotyped rocking — a measure of institution and ward effectiveness. *American Journel of Mental Deficiency*, 1968, **73**, 13-20.

Klaber, M. M. Butterfield, E. C. & Gould, L. J. Responsiveness to social reinforcement among institutionalized retarded children. *American Journal of Mental Deficiency*, 1969, **73**, 890-95.

Kounin, J. Experimental studies of rigidity: I. The measurement of rigidity in normal and feebleminded persons. *Character and Personality*, 1941, **9**, 251-72. (a)

Kounin, J. Experimental studies of rigidity: II. The explanatory power of the concept of rigidity as applied to feeblemindedness. *Character and Personality*, 1941, **9**, 273-82. (b)

Kounin, J. The meaning of rigidity: A reply to Heinz Werner. *Psychological Review*, 1948, **55**, 157-66.

Krishef, C. H. An analysis of some factors in the institutional experience of mentally retarded dischargees from the Owatonna State School that influence their successful or unsuccessful community adjustment. Unpublished manuscript, School of Social Work, University of Minnesota, 1957.

Krugman, M. Some impressions of the Revised Stanford-Binet Scale. *Journal of Educational Psychology*, 1939, **30**, 594-603.

Leahy, A. M. Nature-nurture and intelligence. *Genetic Psychology Monographs*, 1935, **17**, 236-308.

Lewin, K. *A dynamic theory of personality*. New York: McGraw-Hill, 1936.

Lewis, M. Social isolation: A parametric study of its effect on social reinforcement. *Journal of Experimental Child Psychology*, 1965, **2**, 205-18.

Lewis, M. Probability learning in young children: The binary choice paradigm. *Journal of Genetic Psychology*, 1966, **108**, 43-48.

Lewis, M., Wall, A. M. & Aronfreed, J. Developmental change in the relative value of social and nonsocial reinforcement. *Journal of Experimental Psychology*, 1963, **66**, 133-38.

Lucito, L. J. A comparison of independence-conformity behavior of intellectually bright and dull children. Unpublished doctoral dissertation, University of Illinois, 1959.

Luria, A. R. *Problems of higher nervous activity in the normal and nonnormal child*. Moscow: Akad. Pedag. Nauk RSFSR, 1956.

Lyle, J. The effect of an institution environment upon the verbal development of imbecile children. I. Verbal intelligence. *Journal of Mental Deficiency Research*, 1959, 3, 122-28.

Mautner, H. *Mental retardation: Its care, treatment and physiological base*. Elmsford, N. Y.: Pergamon Press, 1959.

McArthur, L. & Zigler, E. Level of satiation on social reinforcers and valence of the reinforcing agent as determinants of social reinforcer effectiveness. *Developmental Psychology*, 1969, 1, 739-46.

McCoy, N. & Zigler, E. Social reinforcer effectiveness as a function of the relationship between child and adult. *Journal of Personality and Social Psychology*, 1965, 1, 604-12.

McKinney, J. P. & Keele, T. Effects of increased mothering on the behavior of severely retarded boys. *American Journal of Mental Deficiency*, 1963, 67, 556-62.

Milgram, N. A. The rationale and irrational in Zigler's motivational approach to mental retardation. *American Journal of Mental Deficiency*, 1969, 73, 527-32.

O'Connor, N. & Hermelin, B. Discrimination and reversal learning in inbeciles. *Journal of Abnormal and Social Psychology*, 1959, 59, 409-13.

Odom, R. D. Problem-solving strategies as a function of age and socio-economic level. *Child Development*, 1967, 38, 753-64.

Penrose, L. S. *The biology of mental defect*. London: Sidgwick & Jackson, 1963.

Plenderleith, M. Discrimination learning and discrimination reversal learning in normal and feebleminded children. *Journal of Genetic Psychology*, 1956, 88, 107-12.

Robinson, H. B. & Robinson, N. M. *A mentally retarded child*. New York: McGraw-Hill, 1965.

Rosen, M., Diggory, J. C., & Werlinsky, B. Goal setting and expectancy of success in institutionalized and noninstitutionalized mental subnormals. *American Journal of Mental Deficiency*, 1966, 71, 249-55.

Rotter, J. B. *Social learning and clinical psychology*. Englewood Cliffs, N. J.: Prentice-Hall, 1954.

Sanders, B., Zigler, E., & Butterfield, E.C. Outer-directedness in the discrimination learning of normal and mentally retarded children. *Journal of Abnormal Psychology*, 1968, 73, 368-75.

Sarason, S. B. *Psychological problems in mental deficiency.* New York: Harper, 1953.

Sarason, S. B., Davidson, K. S., Lighthall, F. F., Waite, R. R., & Ruebush, B. K. *Anxiety in elementary school children.* New York: Wiley, 1960.

Sarason, S. B. & Gladwin, T. Psychological and cultural problems in mental subnormality: A review of research. *Genetic Psychology Monographs*, 1958, 57, 3-290.

Schlanger, B. B. Environmental influences on the verbal output of mentally retarded children. *Journal of Speech and Hearing Disorders*, 1954, 19, 339-45.

Shafter, A. J. Criteria for selecting institutionalized mental defectives for vocational placement. *American Journal of Mental Deficiency*, 1957, 61, 599-616.

Shallenberger, P. & Zigler, E. Rigidity, negative reaction tendencies, and cosatiation effects in normal and feebleminded children. *Journal of Abnormal and Social Psychology*, 1961, 63, 20-26.

Shultz, T. & Zigler, E. Emotional concomitants of visual mastery in infants: The effects of stimulus movement on smiling and vocalizing. *Journal of Experimental Child Psychology*, 1970, 10, 390-402.

Siegel, P. S. & Foshee, J. G. Molar variability in the mentally defective. *Journal of Abnormal and Social Psychology*, 1960, 61, 141-43.

Silverstein, A. B. & Owens, E. P. Factor structure of the social deprivation scale for mongoloid retardates. *American Journal of Mental Deficiency*, 1968, 73, 315-17.

Skeels, H. M., Updegraff, R., Wellman, B. L., & Williams, H. M. A study of environmental stimulation. *University of Iowa Study of Child Welfare*, 1938, 15, No. 4.

Spitz, H. H. Field theory in mental deficiency. In N. R. Ellis (Ed.), *Handbook of mental deficiency.* New York: McGraw-Hill, 1963. Pp. 11-40.

Spitz, R. A. & Wolf, K. M. Anaclitic depression. In Anna Freud *et al.* (Eds.), *The psychoanalytic study of the child.* Vol II. New York: International Universities Press, 1946. Pp. 313-42.

Stevenson, H. W. Social reinforcement with children as a function of CA, sex of *E*, and sex of *S. Journal of Abnormal and Social Psychology*, 1961, 63, 147-54.

Stevenson, H. W. & Fahel, L. The effect of social reinforcement on the performance of institutionalized and noninstitutionalized normal and feebleminded children. *Journal of Personality*, 1961, **29**, 136-47.

Stevenson, H. W. & Weir, M. W. Variables affecting children's performance in a probability learning task. *Journal of Experimental Psychology*, 1959, **57**, 403-12.

Stevenson, H. W. & Weir, M. W. The role of age and verbalization in probability learning. *American Journal of Psychology*, 1963, **76**, 299-305.

Stevenson, H. W. & Zigler, E. Discrimination learning and rigidity in normal and feebleminded individuals. *Journal of Personality*, 1957, **25**, 699-711.

Stevenson, H. W. & Zigler, E. Probability learning in children. *Journal of Experimental Psychology*, 1958, **56**, 185-92.

Tarjan, G. & Benson, F. Report on the pilot study at Pacific Colony. *American Journal of Mental Deficiency*, 1953, **57**, 453-62.

Terrell, G., Jr., Durkin, K., & Wiesley, M. Social class and the nature of the incentive in discrimination learning. *Journal of Abnormal and Social Psychology*, 1959, **59**, 270-72.

Tizard, J. The prevalence of mental subnormality. *Bulletin of the World Health Organization*, 1953, **9**, 423-40.

Tizard, J. Longitudinal and follow-up studies. In A. M. Clarke & A. D. B. Clarke (Eds.), *Mental deficiency: The changing outlook*. New York: Free Press, 1958.

Tolman, E. C. Cognitive maps in rats and men. *Psychological Review*, 1948, **55**, 189-208.

Tuddenham, R. D. The nature and measurement of intelligence. In L. Postman (Ed.), *Psychology in the making*. New York: Knopf, 1962. Pp. 469-525.

Turnure, J. E. Reactions to physical and social distractors by moderately retarded, institutionalized children. *Exceptional Children*, in press.

Turnure, J. E. & Zigler, E. Outer-directedness in the problem-solving of normal and retarded children. *Journal of Abnormal and Social Psychology*, 1964, **69**, 427-36.

Weaver, J. The effects of motivation-hygiene orientation and interpersonal reaction tendencies in intellectually subnormal children. Unpublished doctoral dissertation, George Peabody College for Teachers, 1966.

Weaver, T. R. The incidence of maladjustment among mental defectives in military environment. *American Journal of Mental Deficiency*, 1946, **51**, 238-46.

Weir, M. W. Effects of age and instruction on children's probability learning. *Child Development*, 1962, **33**, 729-35.

Weir, M. W. Developmental changes in problem-solving strategies. *Psychological Review*, 1964, **71**, 473-90.

Wellman, B. L. Guiding mental development. *Childhood Education*, 1938, **15**, 108-12.

White, R. Motivation reconsidered: The concept of competence. *Psychological Review*, 1959, **66**, 297-333.

Windle, C. Prognosis of mental subnormals. *American Journal of Mental Deficiency*, 1962, **66** (Monogr. Suppl. 5).

Wittenborn, J. & Myers, B. *The placement of adoptive children*. Springfield, Ill.: Charles C. Thomas, 1957.

Wolfensberger, W. & Menolascino, F. Basic considerations in evaluating ability of drugs to stimulate cognitive development in retardates. *American Journal of Mental Deficiency*, 1968, **73**, 414-23.

Woodward, M. Early experiences and later social responses of severely subnormal children. *British Journal of Medical Psychology*, 1960, **33**, 123-32.

Yarrow, L. J. Maternal deprivation: Toward an empirical and conceptual reevaluation. *Psychological Bulletin*, 1961, **58**, 459-90.

Yarrow, L. J. Separation from parents during early childhood. In M. L. Hoffman & L. W. Hoffman (Eds.), *Review of child development research*. Vol. I. New York: Russell Sage Foundation, 1964. Pp. 89-137.

Zeaman, D. Discrimination learning in retardates. *Training School Bulletin*, 1959, **56**, 62-67.

Zeaman, D. Review of N. R. Ellis, *International review of research in mental retardation*. (Vol. I.) *Contemporary Psychology*, 1968, **13**, 142-43.

Zeaman, D. & House, B. J. Approach and avoidance in the discrimination learning of retardates. In D. Zeaman *et al.*, *Learning and transfer in mental defectives*. Progress report No. 2, NIMH, USPHS, 1960. Res. Grant M-1099 to University of Connecticut. Pp. 32-70.

Zigler, E. The effect of preinstitutional social deprivation on the performance of feebleminded children. Unpublished doctoral dissertation, University of Texas, 1958.

Zigler, E. Social deprivation and rigidity in the performance of feebleminded children. *Journal of Abnormal and Social Psychology*, 1961, **62**, 413-21.

Zigler, E. Rigidity in the feebleminded. In E. P. Trapp & P. Himelstein (Eds.), *Readings on the exceptional child.* New York: Appleton-Century-Crofts, 1962. Pp. 141-62. (a)

Zigler, E. Social deprivation in familial and organic retardates. *Psychological Reports,* 1962, **10**, 370. (b)

Zigler, E. Rigidity and social reinforcement effects in the performance of institutionalized and noninstitutionalized normal and retarded children. *Journal of Personality,* 1963, **31**, 258-69. (a)

Zigler, E. Social reinforcement, environment and the child. *American Journal of Orthopsychiatry,* 1963, **33**, 614-23. (b)

Zigler, E. The effect of social reinforcement on normal and socially deprived children. *Journal of Genetic Psychology,* 1964, **104**, 235-42.

Zigler, E. Mental retardation: Current issues and approaches. In M. L. Hoffman & L. W. Hoffman (Eds.), *Review of child development research.* Vol. II. New York: Russell Sage Foundation, 1966. Pp. 107-68. (a)

Zigler, E. Motivational determinants in the performance of feebleminded children. *American Journal of Orthopsychiatry,* 1966, **36**, 848-56. (b)

Zigler, E. Research in personality structure in the retardate. In N. R. Ellis (Ed.), *International review of research in mental retardation.* Vol. I. New York: Academic Press, 1966. Pp. 77-108. (c)

Zigler, E., Balla, D., & Butterfield, E. C. A longitudinal investigation of the relationship between preinstitutional social deprivation and social motivation in institutionalized retardates. *Journal of Personality and Social Psychology,* 1968, **10**, 437-45.

Zigler, E. & Butterfield, E. C. Rigidity in the retarded: A further test of the Lewin-Kounin formulation. *Journal of Abnormal Psychology,* 1966, **71**, 224-31.

Zigler, E. & Butterfield, E. C. Motivational aspects of changes in IQ test performance of culturally deprived nursery school children. *Child Development,* 1968, **39**, 1-14.

Zigler, E., Butterfield, E. C., & Capobianco, F. Institutionalization and the effectiveness of social reinforcement: A five- and eight-year follow-up study. *Developmental Psychology,* 1970, **3**, 255-63.

Zigler, E., Butterfield, E. C., & Goff, G. A measure of preinstitutional social deprivation for institutionalized retardates. *American Journal of Mental Deficiency,* 1966, **70**, 873-85.

Zigler, E. & Child, I. Socialization. In G. Lindzey & E. Aronson (Eds.), *The handbook of social psychology.* (2nd ed.) Reading, Mass.: Addison-Wesley, 1969. Pp. 450-589.

Zigler, E. & deLabry, J. Concept-switching in middle-class, lower-class, and retarded children. *Journal of Abnormal and Social Psychology*, 1962, **65**, 267-73.

Zigler, E. & Harter, S. Socialization of the mentally retarded. In D. A. Goslin & D. C. Glass (Eds.), *Handbook of socialization theory and research*. New York: Rand McNally, 1969. Pp. 1065-102.

Zigler, E., Hodgden, L., & Stevenson, H. W. The effect of support on the performance of normal and feebleminded children. *Journal of Personality*, 1958, **26**, 106-22.

Zigler, E. & Kanzer, P. The effectiveness of two classes of verbal reinforcers on the performance of middle- and lower-class children. *Journal of Personality*, 1962, **30**, 157-63.

Zigler, E., Levine, J., & Gould, L. Cognitive processes in the development of children's appreciation of humor. *Child Development*, 1966, **37**, 507-18. (a)

Zigler, E., Levine, J., & Gould, L. The humor response of normal, institutionalized retarded, and noninstitutionalized retarded children. *American Journal of Mental Deficiency*, 1966, **71**, 472-80. (b)

Zigler, E., Levine, J., & Gould, L. Cognitive challenge as a factor in children's humor appreciation. *Journal of Personality and Social Psychology*, 1967, **6**, 332-36.

Zigler, E. & Unell, E. Concept-switching in normal and feebleminded children as a function of reinforcement. *American Journal of Mental Deficiency*, 1962, **66**, 651-57.

Zigler, E. & Williams, J. Institutionalization and the effectiveness of social reinforcement: A three-year follow-up study. *Journal of Abnormal and Social Psychology*, 1963, **66**, 197-205.

Chapter 3

Studies of Psychodiagnostic Errors of Observation as a Contribution Toward a Nondynamic Psychopathology of Everyday Life[1]

Loren J. Chapman

Clinical psychodiagnosticians make errors of observation that are systematic, but yet are not motivated by the needs of the clinician who makes the errors. The errors are instead predictable by formal or structural relationships between ideas or events with which the clinician is dealing. Such errors should be viewed as an aspect of what Freud called the "psychopathology of everyday life," even though the explanation of these errors advanced here is a nondynamic one.

Freud used this phrase, "the psychopathology of everyday life," to refer to errors that normal people frequently make, such as the forgetting of proper names and foreign words, slips of the tongue, errors in reading, and superstitious beliefs. Freud saw unconscious motivation as the core explanation of these phenomena, as well as of neurosis, psychosis, dreams, and the cognitive functioning of so-called "primitive man." Freud also described nondynamic principles to account for the pathways along which motivation acts to produce errors or symptoms. He repeatedly pointed to verbal associative connection as a pathway by which ideas are chosen to be related to one another. An example is the misremembering of a name. The forgotten name, Freud said, often has an associative connection to the erroneous name that is remembered in its place. Freud emphasized, however, that association does not explain the error but is only a pathway by which unconscious need expresses itself. This chapter will show that association acts to produce another important systematic error in cognitive functioning of normal people, and that the nature of these errors is predictable without recourse to motivation as an explanatory principle. This principle might, therefore, be viewed as one building block in a nondynamic psychopathology of everyday life. The paper will focus on the relevance of these errors to difficulties in performing clinical psychodiagnosis.

[1]Portions of this material have previously been published in the *Journal of Verbal Learning and Verbal Behavior* and in the *Journal of Abnormal Psychology*. The author is indebted to Academic Press and to the American Psychological Association for permission to reproduce these materials.

Freud made an immense contribution in pointing out the importance of man's impulse life in shaping his behavior. I believe that this emphasis was, however, excessive in Freud's theory building. Many other writers have made the same criticism, ever since Freud first published his theories. The belief that nondynamic principles may account for many of the phenomena that Freud described has recently been gaining increasing respectability in clinical circles, largely as a result of advances in theory and practice of behavior therapy. However, the possibility that nondynamic principles may be of importance in systematic errors of clinical observation has received much less attention.

Psychodiagnostic Errors

Although the nature of errors in psychodiagnosis has received relatively modest research attention in recent years, the level of accuracy of psychodiagnosis has been investigated at length. One repeated finding has been that psychodiagnostic tests, especially projective tests, are much more difficult for clinicians to use accurately than they commonly believe. Little and Shneidman's (1959) classic study, to take one notable example, showed that expert clinicians using their favorite projective techniques are much less able to make accurate statements about patients than they believe. They performed only slightly better than chance. Other investigators have reported that clinicians are able to use much less information in forming a judgment than they believe, so that increases in the amount of information do not increase accuracy, and that inexperienced diagnosticians are likely to do as well as highly experienced ones. Goldberg (1968) listed 14 studies that demonstrated this latter point and 10 studies that supported the first one. The great bulk of the relevant research evidence is discouraging for traditional psychodiagnostic practice.

In all of the studies just mentioned, the investigators measured the diagnostician's performance primarily in terms of sheer accuracy, and stated their findings in terms of what the diagnosticians failed to do. In contrast, the present chapter will focus on the nature and source of incorrect psychodiagnostic interpretations.

Psychodiagnosticians who are dynamically oriented usually believe that their own systematic errors are interpretable in psychodynamic terms. They believe, in sympathy with the observations of Sigmund Freud, that they themselves, as well as their patients, perceive, remember, and believe partly in response to their emotional needs. They also believe that, by striving to attain awareness of their own dynamics, they can reduce their errors. Freud reported that he was able to scrutinize both his own errors and his neurotic symptoms to discover the emotional needs that lay behind them. By this self-examination, he believed that he brought his cognitions closer to objective reality. Writers on projective testing commonly remind their readers that a projective test may serve as an indicator of the emotional problems of the diagnostician who interprets the test, as well as those of the patient (Eron, 1950; Hammer & Piotrowski, 1953; Masling, 1960; Rotter, 1946; Zubin, Eron, & Schumer, 1965). This concern about motivated error by clinicians is undoubtedly justified.

Freud's discovery that cognitive functioning is distorted by emotional needs has, for many clinicians, brought a semblance of order to clinical chaos. Freud's influence has been so great that psychodiagnosticians have tended to overlook the importance of nonmotivated errors in normal cognition. A number of principles of a nondynamic psychopathology of everyday life have emerged from experimental psychology, although experimental psychologists usually do not term the errors "psychopathology," because they work in a nonclinical research tradition. Obvious examples of systematic errors in normal cognition are the effects of proactive inhibition and retroactive inhibition in forgetting, stimulus generalization and transfer effects in learning, and response biases.

This neglect of nondynamic principles in accounting for the psychopathology of everyday life is paralleled closely by the views of many dynamically oriented clinicians, concerning the schizophrenic thought disorder. Most practicing clinicians whom I have known believe, almost as an article of faith, that each psychotic deviancy in the verbal behavior of schizophrenics is motivated by a need specifically related to the error. Yet the research evidence points out, with unambiguous clarity, that this is not the case. The errors that we call "schizophrenic thought disorder" are predominantly determined by the structural, that is, formal relationships between ideas. For example, when schizophrenics are given a conceptual task in which there is a built-in opportunity for substituting a normal associate for a correct conceptual response, schizophrenics show a far greater propensity to do this than do normal subjects, even when dealing with materials that are emotionally neutral. Very little of the variation in schizophrenic thought disorder is attributable to the emotional impact of the ideas with which the patient is dealing. Several experiments have shown that emotional content affects schizophrenic errors at a statistically significant level, but these effects are small when compared to the massive changes that are readily demonstrable by varying the structural relationships of the words and ideas which one asks the patient to manipulate.

The studies that will be reviewed here deal with one important nondynamic principle of the psychopathology of everyday life that appears to have special importance for the psychodiagnostician who interprets projective tests. The data indicate that the propensity toward this kind of error is not limited to clinical psychodiagnosticians but, instead, seems to be built into most, or, perhaps, all people.

Consider the task of the psychodiagnostician who uses projective tests. He faces an extremely large array of test responses from which he attempts to infer a description of the patient who produced those responses. He must have some basis for inferring a given characteristic of a patient from a given kind of test response, or from a given pattern of test responses. What can he use as a basis for such inferences? First of all, of course, he can read the manuals of the various projective tests and learn what the experts say concerning the characteristics of patients who produce each kind of test response. He can also rely on what his teachers and colleagues have told him that they have observed. The seasoned, experienced clinician, however, expects to rely on his own clinical experience. Most diagnosticians value clinical experience very highly. They believe that one must see many patients, together with their test responses, in order to learn which kinds of test responses are produced by various kinds of patients. The psychodiagnostician then feels able to rely on his accumulated clinical observations in order to make statements concerning patients after seeing their test responses.

The task of accumulating clinical experience is largely one of observing two classes of events. One class consists of characteristics of patients, and the other of characteristics of test responses. The clinician attempts to observe and remember correlations between these two classes of events. The term "correlation" is not intended here to refer to any particular statistical measure, such as the Pearson product moment correlation coefficient, but is, instead, intended to refer merely to concomitance of events.

The observation of correlations between classes of events is a central task in everyone's life. Everyone must base many of his decisions, from moment to moment, on such accumulated observations. Consider, for example, such correlational statements as these:

> When there are clouds in the sky, it is likely to rain.
> Eating rapidly may produce indigestion.
> Sitting in a draft is often followed by catching a cold.

If the observer is a clinician, he is likely to store in his memory such correlational statements as:

> People who have a rich fantasy life produce, on the Rorschach, more movement responses than people with an impoverished fantasy life.
> People who are concerned about their intellectual functioning are more likely, on the Draw-A-Person Test, to draw unusual heads than are people without such concerns.

It is clear, however, that observations of this kind are difficult to make with accuracy. Systematic errors, as well as random ones, frequently appear. One very common systematic error is the report of a correlation that is not warranted by the objective facts. Different observers often agree as to the existence of such a correlation even though it is incorrect.

I have proposed the term "illusory correlation" for the report by an observer of a correlation between two classes of events which, in reality, (1) are not correlated, or (2) are correlated to a lesser extent than reported, or (3) are correlated in the opposite direction than that which is reported.

In my laboratory, my colleagues and I have accumulated considerable evidence that one source of systematic error in the report of correlations is associative connection between classes of events. This chapter will review evidence that events which have a verbal associative connection are seen as correlated in their occurrence when, in fact, they are not. Associative connection refers here simply to the phenomenon that one idea tends to call to mind another idea. For example, the word "mountain" tends to call to mind "top"; the word "black" tends to call to mind "white."

We will first look at some of the evidence accumulated in laboratory situations in which pairs of words were the stimuli. Next will be some studies in which projective test materials were used as stimuli.

Other Names for the Phenomena of Illusory Correlation

Phenomena that may be formulated in terms of illusory correlation have been given a variety of names. They have often been called superstition or folklore. An example might be the report that birth deformity is correlated with the mother's looking at a snake or a deformed person. Another example is the report that one's luck is better when carrying a good luck piece.

When the observers are professional people, such as physicians and psychologists, such phenomena are often called "errors in clinical observation." Many clinicians who use the Draw-A-Person Test often report that they have observed that those patients who show paranoid behavior also show more elaboration of the eye in their drawings. Yet four separate studies have failed to substantiate this observation by a counting of the relevant phenomena (Fisher & Fisher, 1950; Holzberg & Wexler, 1950; Reznikoff & Nicholas, 1958; Ribler, 1957). A marginal exception to these uniformly negative findings is an investigation by Griffith and Peyman (1959). These investigators selected, from the drawings of 745 patients, the extreme 3% on elaboration of either the eye or the ear, or both. This extreme group differed from an unselected group of patients on ideas of reference.

The great bulk of evidence concerning the correlation between symptoms of patients and drawing characteristics has disconfirmed popular clinical beliefs. Swensen (1957) reviewed the DAP research literature concerned with the validity of Machover's (1949) principles of DAP interpretation and concluded that almost all were unsupported. In his more recent review, Swensen (1968) concluded that only overall goodness of drawing, and other qualities of drawings that reflect overall quality, are clearly related to the absence of pathology. He found almost no evidence for relationships between specific content or characteristics of drawings and specific characteristics of patients. Roback (1968) reviewed much of the same evidence and also concluded that most of the published studies failed to support Machover's hypotheses. He believed, however, there were too few well-designed investigations to reach a final conclusion. If many clinicians agree that they observe relationships not supported by relevant data, one might suspect that their reported observations are illusory correlations which are both systematic in direction and shared by many observers.

Some instances of illusory correlations have, at some times in history, been viewed as superstition but, at other times, as errors in clinical observation. For many centuries it was believed, presumably on the basis of clinical observation, that both epileptic fits and outbursts of psychotic behavior occur more often at the full of the moon. For many centuries in Europe, this was regarded as sound medical observation and the term, "lunacy", bears witness to the former prevalence of the belief. Only a few present-day physicians and other professional workers still believe in the correlation, and such people occasionally publish clinical reports of an ancedotal nature in support of the hypothesis (Ravitz, 1952, 1953, 1955). However, most professional people regard the belief as a superstition and careful research has consistently failed to substantiate the observations (Chapman, 1961; Temkin, 1945).

The practice of magic, as in nonliterate societies, is usually defended by its practitioners on the grounds that they have observed that the magical ritual is correlated with the desired effects. Although the belief in magic seems ridiculously naive to modern Western man, the tendency toward the kind of errors of observation which are necessary for such continued belief may be stronger in us than we would like to think. The natives of Timor report that killing a white pig is more often followed by sunshine and that killing a black pig is more often followed by rain; the Hopi and Pueblo Indians perform their famous rain dances to bring rain; some of my friends report that washing a car will surely produce rain.

Many errors of observation necessary for the perpetuation of racial and religious prejudice may also be conceptualized in terms of illusory correlation. Prejudiced persons often report observing strong relationships between race or religion and certain undesirable personal characteristics, although more careful investigation may fail to support the observation.

Some related phenomena have sometimes been called the "halo effect," especially when the evaluation is a positive one. The halo effect refers to the tendency of judges to rate a person high on one socially valued characteristic, if they rate him high on other valued characteristics. For example, Thorndike (1920) reported that for groups of army officers who rated one another, the correlations between ratings for characteristics such as intelligence and physique were far higher than warranted by the facts.

All of the above phenomena indicate that illusory correlation is an extremely prevalent error, and that different observers often report the same unwarranted correlation. It seems likely that the principles which would account for the formation of illusory correlation in one of these subject matter areas may account for it in other areas. The same psychological principles may account for illusory correlation in such apparently divergent areas as superstition, primitive magic, errors in clinical observation, social prejudice, and halo effect.

The most immediately obvious and widely accepted source of illusory correlation is, of course, prior belief. That is, people report that they observe correlations of a sort in which they already believe. Although this may be a potent source of illusory correlation, prior belief cannot account for the origin of the belief in the correlation in the first place. It seems likely that the origin of such beliefs can best be sought in terms of the characteristics of the stimulus events which are erroneously perceived as correlated, or in terms of the observers' responses to the stimulus events.

The Associative Basis of Much Illusory Correlation

One such characteristic appears to be verbal associative connection between the ideas representing stimulus events. Associative connection usually is formed if the events are similar to one another, or if they are experienced in contiguity to one another. The literature on primitive magic, superstition, and folklore indicates that similarity of objects and past contiguity of objects are powerful variables in producing illusory correlation. Many omens and most imitative or homeopathic magic are predicated on a correlation in the frequency of occurrence of similar events, as described at great length by Frazer (1935) and as discussed by Freud (1938). Frazer, in his classic anthropological work, *The Golden Bough*, described hundreds of magical practices that are predicated on the principle that similar events are correlated in their occurrence, or that objects that have been related to one another in the past change in a correlated fashion. Sometimes the stimulus dimension is one of physical similarity. In the use of voodoo dolls, a doll resembling one's enemy is injured and the practitioners report observing a correlation between injury to the doll and injury to the victim. In other magical practices, the similarity is more one of analogy between events. For example, natives of both Java and Central America have intercourse in the fields in order to stimulate growth of the crops (Vol. II, p. 98). In many rain-producing rituals, rain is imitated in order to produce rain. For all such magical practices, the practitioners report observing a correlation between their ritual and the desired event.

Superstitions, likewise, often consist of an illusory correlation that is apparently based on an analogy between two events. Radford and Radford (1949) described an observational report, which is found in Aristotle, Shakespeare, and Dickens, that deaths mostly occur at the ebbing of the tide. In this belief, there appears to be a similarity or analogy between the ebbing of the tide and the ebbing of life. Radford and Radford state that this belief is still widely held both among seamen and inhabitants of the coastal areas of England.

Contagious magic, to use Frazer's term, is based on the principle that things that have been in contact with one another continue to be in contact. The magician may, for example, attempt to injure a person by destroying an article of his clothing or, more beneficently, attempt to cure a knife wound by cleaning the knife that caused the wound. He believes that the events that happen in relation to the one object also happen to the other.

Frazier concluded that the two central principles of the magician's logic are two different misapplications of the association of ideas. He believed that homeopathic magic is founded on the association of ideas by similarity, and that contagious magic is founded on the association of ideas by contiguity.

Freud (1938) relied heavily on Frazer's work in developing his own theory of primitive magic, but objected that "the association theory of magic merely explains the paths that magic travels and not its essential nature." Freud believed that he found its essential nature in the "omnipotence of thoughts," that is, the belief that thinking a thing or, more importantly, wishing a thing, has the power to make it happen. Freud believed that he found this principle not only in primitive magic, but also in the thinking of children and in the symptoms of neurotic and psychotic patients.

I believe that Freud was mistaken in his belief that dynamic principles are necessary to account for the tendency to mistake the order of ideas for the order of nature. This chapter will present laboratory studies that explored the report of a correlation between the occurrences of associatively related ideas. In these laboratory situations, it is almost impossible to imagine that the nature of each erroneously reported correlation is determined by a wish of the observer.

Illusory Correlation in the Observation of Pairs of Words

The purpose of the first investigation was to produce illusory correlation and to investigate some of the variables that account for its occurrence. Hypotheses concerning these variables were drawn from the examples above. The leap is broad from these complicated behaviors in diverse settings to the manipulations of an experiment. It seemed desirable, nevertheless, to study illusory correlation in controlled experiments in order to determine what variables produce it.

In the first two experiments to be reported here, illusory correlation based on similarity or associative connection was investigated using words as stimuli. In the first study, the effect of semantic similarity in producing illusory correlation was studied. It was difficult, however, to vary degree of semantic similarity without, at the same time, varying associative connection because, as discussed above, similar events tend to call one another to mind. Objective measurement has demonstrated the great strength of the relationship. Haagen (1949), using ratings on 400 pairs of adjectives that varied on semantic similarity, found a correlation of .90 between similarity of meaning and closeness of associative connection.

The method used in both of these studies was that of presenting to the S a series of pairs of words printed on pages of a booklet (Experiment 1) or projected on a screen (Experiment 2). At each stimulus presentation, a single pair was shown, one word on the left and one on the right. The words were taken from two sets, one set being reserved for presentation on the left hand side and the other set for presentation on the right hand side, with every possible pairing of left hand words with right hand words appearing equally often. The S was told before viewing the word pairs that his task was to observe and report how often each word was paired with each other word. Actually, there was no true correlation between the occurrence of any left hand word and any right hand word. However, there were relationships of high similarity or high strength associative connection between some left hand words and some right hand words. It was hypothesized that the Ss would err by reporting words of high similarity or high associative connection as correlated in their occurrence.

Experiment 1 — Word Pairs Presented in Booklets

The following two sets of words were selected:

Left Hand Words	Right Hand Words
worldly	puny
peaceful	blotchy
irksome	fiscal
rounded	hybrid
	tranquil
	sterile

The four words on the left and the six words on the right yielded 24 pairs. A single one of these pairs, "peaceful-tranquil," was chosen to be of both high semantic similarity and high strength associative connection, while the remaining 23 were low on both of these variables.

Ratings for similarity of meaning and for associative connection, by a group of 36 judges, confirmed that this was the case.

Experimental task. Booklets were prepared with a single pair of words on each page, with both words on a single line. Altogether there were 240 pairings which were presented in random order, the only restriction on randomness being that each of the 24 pairs appeared 10 times. The Ss were 41 students in an undergraduate course in experimental psychology.

The booklets were presented to the Ss with the following instructions:

> This is an experiment on accuracy of observation. I am going to give each of you a booklet to look through. On each page there will be two words. Several words will be used in various pairings on different pages. When you are done, we are going to ask you some questions about which words appeared together most often. Look through the booklet as quickly as you can, but be sure to notice which words are paired together on each page.

It is seen that in this design there was no actual correlation between the occurrence of any left hand word and any right hand word. The prediction was that, contrary to this objective reality, the Ss would report a correlation between the occurrence of "peaceful" and "tranquil." That is, they would report that when "peaceful" occurred on the left, "tranquil" occurred on the right more often than the other right hand words.

After the Ss had completed their inspection of the booklets they were given a questionnaire containing items of the following format:

> When the word "worldly" appeared, estimate the percentage of those times that it was paired with each of the following:
>
> _____ puny
> _____ blotchy
> _____ fiscal
> _____ hybrid
> _____ sterile
> _____ tranquil

TOTAL 100%

A similar item was presented for each of the other three left hand words and, in each item, the six right hand words were listed in the same order. Each percentage value listed by the S is termed here his "reported co-occurrence" of that right hand word with the given left hand word. Illusory correlation is measured by the disparity between the reported co-occurrence and the objectively correct co-occurrence.

Results. For the "peaceful-tranquil" pair, the reported co-occurrence was 23.5%, that is, when the word "peaceful" occurred, the average S reported "tranquil" as occurring 23.5% of the time. The objectively correct co-occurrence for each pair was, of course, 16 2/3%. The other 23 reported co-occurrence values were lower than this, ranging from 12.6% to 20.6%, with a mean of 16.36%.

A t-test was computed between the reported percentage for "peaceful-tranquil" and the objectively accurate percentage of 16.7%. The difference was highly significant ($t = 3.14, p < .01$).

The data were examined with regard to the feasibility of two alternative explanations of the results. If a S believed that "tranquil" occurred more often than any other right hand word, regardless of which left hand word was present, the reported co-occurrence of "peaceful-tranquil" would be elevated without the effect being due to the semantic similarity or associative connection of "tranquil" to "peaceful." However, this is clearly not the case since the reported co-occurrences of "tranquil" with the other three left hand words were all slightly less than 16 2/3%.

Experiment 1 indicates that high similarity and/or associative connection produces illusory correlation. However, it does not make it possible to separate the effects of similarity from the effects of associative strength, since "peaceful-tranquil" differ from the other pairs both in their high similarity of meaning and in their high associative strength.

Experiment 2 — Word Pairs Presented on a Film Strip

Experiment 2 was designed primarily to test the effects of associative strength in illusory correlation, with similarity ranging from moderate to low. The study used pairs of words with high associative strength, some of which also were fairly similar in meaning, and others not at all similar. This experiment was also designed to test for the influence of three other variables in producing illusory correlation:

1. Length of series, i.e., the number of pairings presented.
2. Number of prior experiences with other such series of word pairs.
3. Distinctiveness of atypically long words.

The first two variables were studied primarily to determine whether illusory correlation is a sufficiently robust phenomenon that will persist with varying degrees of exposure to relevant stimuli.

The third variable was studied as a source of illusory correlation other than associative strength. In an earlier exploratory study, it appeared that when a single left hand word and a single right hand word were noticeably longer than all the other words, an illusory correlation was formed between these two long words, apparently as a function of the greater distinctiveness of long words in a series of shorter words. One of the aims of Experiment 2 was to investigate this phenomenon more systematically.

Procedure. Three parallel series of word pairs were designed. As in Experiment 1, two words appeared at each stimulus presentation, one on the left and one on the right. However, in Experiment 2, word pairs were photographed on a film strip and projected on a screen. This was done to make it possible to control the length of time each pair was exposed. The frames, each of which presented one pair of words, were changed every two seconds.

In each series, there were four words used on the left and three words used on the right. The sets of words used on the left and on the right in the three series are shown below:

Series A		Series B		Series C	
Left	Right	Left	Right	Left	Right
boat	tiger	door	head	clock	butter
lion	eggs	hat	fork	bread	foot
bacon	notebook	knife	magazine	hand	sidewalk
blossoms		building		envelope	

As seen above, 2 of the 12 pairs of each series had a high strength associative connection and the other 10 pairs had low strength associative connection. Also, one word used on the left and one word used on the right were three or four letters longer than any other word. In addition, one word used on the left was a filler word in that it neither was of atypical length nor had a high strength associate on the right. Unlike Experiment 1, the word pairs with high strength association were not highly similar in meaning. As in Experiment 1, ratings by a group of judges confirmed the accuracy of these statements concerning similarity and associative connection.

Each of the three series was prepared in three different lengths so that each of the 12 possible pairs was presented equally often in the first 48 pairings, in the first 120, and in the entire 240 pairings.

Three groups of Ss were tested. Each group received three successive testings within a single hour, and received in its three testings all three series and all three lengths of series. The order of presentation of the three series and the three lengths of series were counterbalanced across the three groups of Ss.

Each of the three series appeared equally often in the three ordinal testings (i.e., first, second or third testing) and each was presented once for each of the three lengths of series. Also, each of the three lengths of series appeared once in each of the three testings. This design made it possible to observe the effects of series, of series length, and of ordinal testing of the series, independently of the effects of one another.

After each series, the S was given a questionnaire which inquired about co-occurrence of the words. It contained four items, one for each left hand word of that series, all in the following format:

When the word "lion" appeared, estimate the percentage of those times that it was paired with each of the following:

_____ tiger

_____ eggs

_____ notebook

TOTAL 100%

Subjects. The Ss were 163 students from a large introductory psychology course, divided among the three groups.

Results.

Presence of illusory correlation. Table I shows the mean reported co-occurrence at each of the three testings for the nine word pairs for which illusory correlation was predicted. As seen there, the three series were fairly comparable on these values.

The correct co-occurrence in each case was, of course, 33 1/3%. The presence of illusory correlation was tested for each of the nine word pairs by comparing the obtained scores with the correct value of 33 1/3%. A double-tailed large sample t-test was used, pooling the three testings.

The difference was significant for each of the six pairs with high strength associative connection (z = 3.45 or larger, $p < .001$ in each case). Thus illusory correlation was found for word pairs of high strength associative connection but low similarity of meaning (hat-head; bread-butter).

The reported co-occurrence of each of the other two right hand words with each of the left hand associate words was, in every case, less than the objectively correct value of 33 1/3%. This is not surprising because of the restriction that the percentage values for the three right hand words total 100% in each case. The mean co-occurrence between the left hand filler words and the right hand associative words was 32.5, close to the correct value of 33 1/3%.

Since several of these pairs of words with high associative connection had low similarity of meaning, these findings clearly demonstrate that the occurrence of illusory correlation on the basis of associative connection is not dependent on similarity.

For each of the three pairs of atypically long words, the mean reported co-occurrence was also higher than the correct value of 33 1/3% (z = 5.40 or larger, $p < .001$) in each case. This is interpreted as occurring on the basis of the distinctiveness of the long words. However, one might suspect that the high reported co-occurrence of the pair of atypically long words in each series arose as the result of an erroneous observation that the long word on the right hand side occurred more often than the other two right hand words, regardless of which word appeared on the left. This would result if distinctive

Table I

The Mean Reported Co-occurrence at Each of the Three Testings for the Nine Pairs of Words for which Illusory Correlation was Predicted

	First Testing	Second Testing	Third Testing
Series A			
lion — tiger	41.3	37.4	33.8
bacon — eggs	46.7	37.0	35.8
blossoms — notebook	47.0	45.9	43.6
Series B			
hat — head	43.7	36.3	37.9
knife — fork	40.2	34.2	35.8
building — magazine	44.8	43.6	39.0
Series C			
bread — butter	43.3	40.8	36.4
hand — foot	39.1	39.3	34.2
envelope — sidewalk	41.5	40.0	37.3

stimuli are seen as occurring more often than nondistinctive stimuli. This possibility was investigated by examining the reported co-occurrence of the long right hand word in each series with the left hand filler word. The mean values, pooling the three testings, were "boat-notebook," 32.6; "door-magazine," 35.9; and "clock-sidewalk," 36.7. These values differed significantly from 33 1/3% for "door-magazine," $z = 2.33$, $p < .05$, and for "clock-sidewalk," $z = 2.78, p < .01$. This indicates that the erroneously high reported co-occurrence of the pairs of long words may have been inflated by an error of seeing each long right hand word as having a heightened frequency. In order to determine whether the long pairs showed illusory correlation beyond that which might be attributed to such an effect, the reported co-occurrence of each of the long right hand words with the long left hand word was compared with the reported co-occurrence of the long right hand word with the left hand filler word by means of a direct difference t-test. It was found that the reported co-occurrence was significantly greater for "blossoms-notebook" than for "boat-notebook" ($t = 8.25, p < .001$) and was greater for "building-magazine" than for "door-magazine" ($t = 4.26, p <$

.001), and tended to be greater for "envelope-sidewalk" than for "clock-sidewalk" ($t = 1.85, p < .07$). These results indicate that illusory correlation took place for the pairs of long words over and above that which might be attributed to the Ss' attributing excessive frequency to each alone.

As seen in Table I, the amount of illusory correlation declined across successive testings. Combining word pairs from the three series, the mean reported co-occurrence for the associate pairs was found to have dropped from the first testing (42.30) to the second (37.66) and from the second to the third testing (35.64). An analysis of variance showed that this decline was significant ($F = 17.65, df = 2,324, p < .01$).

Similarly, the mean reported co-occurrence declined across successively presented series for the long words. The values here for the first, second, and third testings were 44.36, 43.09, and 40.15, respectively, ($F = 3.56, df = 2,324, p < .05$). The reason for these declines is unknown. However, they may indicate that some Ss "caught on" to the nature of the experiment as they progressed through the three series, or they may be attributable to fatigue and lowered attention. It is also possible that these declines represent a genuine improvement in handling the task as a function of practice.

Length of series and amount of illusory correlation. There was a small but significant variation in illusory correlation for the associate pairs between the three lengths of series. The mean illusory correlation scores for the three lengths of series were 38.35 (short), 40.16 (medium), and 37.09 (long). The three values differed significantly, as determined by analysis of variance ($F = 3.33, df = 2,324, p < .05$). For the pairs of long words, the values were 42.91 (short), 41.79 (medium), and 42.89 (long), and they did not differ significantly ($F = .31, df = 2,324, p > .05$).

Discussion. The present two experiments clearly demonstrate that illusory correlation occurs on the basis of associative connection between stimuli, and that this effect is not dependent on similarity of events. It would be difficult to investigate the converse possibility that illusory correlation occurs in response to semantic similarity, independent of associative connection. As has been pointed out by Bastian (1961), there are very few word pairs of high semantic similarity but low strength associative connection as measured by a word association test. It seems likely that the few high similarity-low association word pairs which do occur may be shown by more sensitive measures to have a stronger associative connection than most low similarity pairs. A rating scale measure of associative connection, such as was used in this study, appears to be more sensitive to small differences in strength among weak associates than a word association test.

Experiment 2 also showed clearly the occurrence of illusory correlation for atypically long words in a list. This was interpreted as occurring on the basis of the distinctiveness of the long words. It is possible, of course, that this dimension could instead be viewed as one of physical similarity. The role of distinctiveness in producing illusory correlation can best be resolved by further research in which other varieties of distinctiveness are manipulated. Experiment 2 also showed that illusory correlation occurs with several different lengths of series, and does not disappear with repeated testings. It does, however, diminish with successive testings using pairs of words as stimuli.

Erroneous Psychodiagnostic Observations

The next several studies used clinical materials in designs closely analogous to those of the above two studies of illusory correlation in the observation of pairs of words. These next studies used laboratory approximations of the task of the beginning clinician who observes the responses of patients to a test in order to discover the kinds of test responses that are made by patients with each of several different kinds of symptoms. The purpose of these studies was to determine the extent of illusory correlation in such observations, to investigate the basis of such errors, and the conditions under which they occur. The DAP was chosen because although most of its popular uses appear to lack validity, it is a widely used test. Sundberg (1961) found in a survey of clinical practice that it is second only to the Rorschach in frequency of usage.

Machover (1949) described the clinical meaning of the DAP almost entirely in terms of clinical correlates of various drawing characteristics. She also mentioned that the patients' verbalizations about the drawings may be useful, but she regarded such data as "of only supplemental significance" (p. 29). The present studies are concerned with illusory correlation between patients' symptoms and their drawings and are not concerned with the patients' verbalizations.

The method of the present studies was to present to naive observers a series of DAP drawings, each drawing being arbitrarily paired with contrived statements about the symptoms of the alleged patient who drew it. Six different statements of symptoms were used and each was attached to several different drawings. The observers were asked to inspect the drawings and the symptom statements describing the patients in order to discover what kinds of drawings were made by patients with each symptom. In looking through the paired drawings and symptom statements, the observers were accumulating "clinical experience" as to the meanings of various aspects of DAP performance. However, in all but one of these experiments (Experiment 4), the drawings and the symptom statements were paired in such a way that there was no relationship between the occurrence of any symptom and any drawing characteristic which is viewed as its correlate in conventional clinical practice.

The hypothesis was that the naive observers would "rediscover" in the drawings the widely accepted correlates of the six symptoms, despite the fact that these relationships did not exist in the task materials. If many of the naive observers should report the same correlates, one must infer shared systematic errors. If these should be the same correlates that clinicians commonly report on the basis of their clinical practice, one might suspect that the clinicians also show these same systematic errors.

Subjects used in the seven studies. All of the Ss were students in an introductory psychology course, except for Experiment 5, in which 23 of the 41 Ss were from more advanced undergraduate psychology courses. No S served in more than one study.

All Ss were naive concerning the DAP. In order to be certain of their naiveté, the examiner gave each S a brief questionnaire which asked whether or not he "had heard" of the DAP before and, if he had, to list one drawing characteristic together with its interpretation. The Ss who showed any indication of prior acquaintance with the DAP were dropped from the sample; this procedure was necessary for a total of 18 Ss in the seven studies.

Experiment 1 — Associatively Based Illusory Correlation in Clinical Practice and in the Laboratory

Method. Six symptom statements were used for pairing with drawings. The six symptom statements were:

1. He is worried about how manly he is.
2. He is suspicious of other people.
3. He is worried about how intelligent he is.
4. He is concerned with being fed and taken care of by other people.
5. He has had problems of sexual impotence.
6. He is very worried that people are saying bad things about him.

Preliminary survey of practicing psychodiagnosticians. Before testing naive observers, it was first necessary to learn the characteristics of the drawings that practicing psychodiagnosticians report they have observed to be correlated with each of the six symptoms. An anonymous questionnaire was used to elicit this information from clinicians. For each of the six symptoms or emotional problems, the questionnaire presented an item of the following form:

He is worried about how manly he is.

The pictures drawn by such men would more often be characterized by

1. . . . .
2. . . . .

The clinician was instructed to assume in each case that the patient was a man who drew a picture of a man.

The questionnaire did not ask for the clinician's name, but it asked for his academic degrees and the year each was obtained, the number of years of his psychodiagnostic experience, and the extent to which he used the DAP. It also asked the clinician whether he found the test useful for discovering the emotional problems of patients.

The questionnaire was circulated primarily by mailing several copies, with return envelopes, to each of a number of clinical psychologists who were interested in psychodiagnosis and who worked with other clinical psychologists. Almost all recipients of the questionnaires were in widely known departments in hospitals, clinics, or universities which have large psychology training programs, either in the form of intern training or graduate teaching. The recipients were asked to distribute the questionnaire with return envelope to each of their colleagues who were active in diagnostic testing. About two-thirds of the questionnaires were returned, 67 in all. Of the 67 respondents, 44 answered the questions fully and also said that they found the test useful. Only these 44 are included in the present analysis. Most of them said that they used the DAP regularly as part of a larger battery of tests. All but 10 of the 44 held the Ph.D. degree, and the group reported a mean of 8.4 years of psychodiagnostic experience.

The clinicians' responses concerning the drawing characteristics which are correlates of each of the six symptoms were tabulated, combining similar statements of drawing characteristics. For example, a single category was used for muscular, broad-shouldered, manly, or athletic builds. About 35 such categories were used.

The choice of how many of these categories of drawing characteristics to report is a somewhat arbitrary one. The decision here is to report all those which were listed by 15% or more of the clinicians as a correlate of at least one symptom statement. A total of 14 drawing characteristics met this criterion, and 6 of these 14 met the criterion for two different symptom statements. For example, "broad-shouldered, muscular figures" met the criterion for the symptoms of both impotence (25%) and worry about manliness (80%). These 14 drawing characteristics may be found in Table II (the first 14 characteristics listed there), together with the percentage of the clinicians who gave each one for each symptom statement. Most, if not all, of the most popular correlates were ones that were either specifically listed by Machover (1949) or are consistent with the principles of interpretation that she advanced.

One of the purposes of this research was to compare these reports, made by clinicians on the basis of their clinical practice, with similar observations by naive observers who were shown randomly paired drawings and symptom statements. The expectation was that the naive judges would erroneously report observing, in such contrived clinical materials, the same relationships between drawing characteristics and symptoms that clinicians reported observing in their diagnostic practice.

Construction of task materials. A set of 45 drawings were collected from psychotic patients at a state hospital and from graduate students in clinical psychology. High quality Xerox reproductions of each drawing were obtained in order to produce multiple sets of the stimulus materials. Printed on the same sheet of paper as each drawing was a pair of statements concerning the alleged symptoms of the patient who made the drawing, for example:

> The man who drew this
> 1. is suspicious of other people.
> 2. is worried about how manly he is.

These pairs of symptom statements were taken from the six symptoms for which the practicing psychodiagnosticians had listed DAP correlates. The pairs of symptom statements were assigned to the drawings so that each symptom statement appeared once with each of 15 drawings.

Three parallel forms (Forms A, B, and C) of the task were constructed, all using the one set of 45 drawings and six symptom statements, by systematically reassigning the symptom statements among the drawings. This pairing was done in such a way that, pooling the three forms, each of the six symptom statements appeared only once with each of the 45 drawings. Thus, by definition, each drawing characteristic occurred as often with one symptom statement as another.

Appropriate precautions were also taken to prevent, within each form, any differential relationship between the occurrence of each symptom and any drawing characteristic which clinicians reported as its correlate. This control was achieved by rank ordering the drawings on the characteristics previously selected for popularity among clinicians, and then by pairing the symptom statement equally often with the drawings having each of various degrees of possession of the drawing characteristic. For example, the symptom statement, "He is worried about how intelligent he is," was paired as often with drawings having small heads as with large or medium sized heads. As will be discussed later, the design provided a convenient internal check on any possible inadequacy of this balancing which would account for any of the reports by observers, concerning correlates of symptoms. This possibility could be checked simply by comparing the three forms as to the content of these reports, and the comparison showed that the balancing was successful.

Procedure. There were 108 Ss divided into three groups (Ns = 34, 38, and 36), each of which received a different one of the three forms of the task.

The Ss were tested in groups. The experimenter (E) first presented a brief description of the DAP and its clinical use, explaining that psychologists

Table II

Percentage of Clinicians and Naive Observers Reporting Various Drawing Characteristics as Accompanying the Six Symptom Statements

Drawing Characteristic	Manliness		Suspicious		Intelligence		Fed and cared for		Impotence		Say bad things	
	Clinician	Observer	Clinician	Observer	Clinician	Observer	Clinician	Observer	Clinician	Observer	Clinician	Observer
1. Broad shoulders, muscular, manly	80	76	0	6	0	8	0	12	25	31	0	6
2. Feminine, child-like	23	22	7	12	2	11	32	39	23	25	11	13
3. Hair distinctive	23	13	2	2	2	8	0	1	11	6	0	3
4. Eyes atypical	0	0	91	58	0	6	0	3	2	2	43	26
5. Ears atypical	0	0	55	6	0	3	0	0	2	0	64	7
6. Facial expression atypical	0	17	18	44	2	21	2	21	2	14	18	52
7. Head large or emphasized	0	5	0	13	82	55	2	7	0	3	9	10
8. Detailed drawing	20	8	2	6	34	13	0	3	7	3	2	6
9. Mouth emphasis	0	0	7	5	0	1	68	8	2	1	5	5

Table II (Cont.)

Percentage of Clinicians and Naive Observers Reporting Various Drawing Characteristics as Accompanying the Six Symptom Statements

Drawing Characteristic	Manliness		Suspicious		Intelligence		Fed and cared for		Impotence		Say bad things	
	Clinician	Observer	Clinician	Observer	Clinician	Observer	Clinician	Observer	Clinician	Observer	Clinician	Observer
10. Passive posture, outstretched arms	5	4	2	8	0	2	36	21	2	2	0	8
11. Buttons	0	0	0	0	0	0	23	1	0	0	0	0
12. Sexual area elaborated	14	5	0	0	0	0	0	0	55	8	0	0
13. Sexual area deemphasized	0	0	0	0	0	0	0	0	18	27	0	0
14. Phallic nose, limbs	9	0	0	0	0	0	0	0	23	2	0	0
15. Fat	0	2	0	1	0	0	7	16	0	4	0	1

make interpretations about patients' emotional problems from the nature of their drawings. However, no examples of relevant drawing characteristics were offered.

The *E* then instructed *S*s as follows:

> Now we want to test your powers of judgment and observation. I'm going to show you some drawings made by men with various emotional problems. Together with each drawing you will find two statements that describe the emotional problems of the man who made the drawing. Many of the men have some of the same problems. Please study the pictures and the statements carefully because, when you are through, I am going to ask you about the characteristics of the drawings that were made by men with each kind of problem.

Each *S* saw each drawing for 30 seconds. After all of the *S*s had seen all 45 pictures, they were given questionnaires which contained items of the following format:

> Some of the pictures were drawn by men with the following problem:

He is worried about how manly he is.

> The pictures drawn by these men were more often characterized by
> 1. ....
> 2. ....
> 3. ....

Five additional items of a format identical to the above were built around the other five symptom statements.

Results. The responses of *S*s receiving each of the three forms of the task were tabulated and were found, as expected, to be highly comparable. (The comparability of the three forms will be discussed in greater detail below.) Therefore, they were combined for purposes of the main analysis of results.

In all, there are 15 drawing characteristics listed in Table II, although two of them ("buttons" and "phallic nose or limbs") seldom occurred for the experimental *S*s. For each of the remaining 13, a Cochran's Q analysis showed that the distribution among the six symptoms differed from chance ($p < .01$, in each case). This finding means that the different *S*s agreed above chance on which symptom occurred with each drawing characteristic.

Of central interest is the degree of similarity between the clinicians and experimental *S*s in the drawing characteristics that were listed as correlates of each symptom. It is seen in Table II that for each of the 15 drawing characteristics, the symptom for which the clinicians most often reported it as a correlate was the same symptom for which the naive observers most often reported it (with the exception of a single tie). For example, both the clinicians and naive observers reported broad-shouldered, muscular figures more often as a correlate of the symptom, "He is worried about how manly he is", than for any other of the six symptoms, and both groups reported drawings with atypical eyes more often for the symptom, "He is suspicious of other people," than for any other symptom.

One may also examine the data of Table II from the opposite starting point; that is, taking one symptom at a time, one may compare the clinicians and experimental Ss as to which drawing characteristic they most often reported as a correlate of that symptom. From this point of view, the agreement was again impressive, although imperfect. For three of the six symptoms (numbers 1, 2, and 3), the two groups most often listed the same one of the 15 drawing characteristics. For each of the six symptoms, the two groups had in common two of the three drawing characteristics that they listed most frequently as its correlate.

It is clear that the experimental Ss showed massive illusory correlation and that the illusory correlates that they reported showed a remarkable similarity to the correlates that clinicians reported from their clinical practice.

Comparability of forms. As mentioned above, the design made it possible to rule out true relationships as a source of the correlates reported, simply by comparing these reports for the three forms. If any relationship was a true one for one form, it would necessarily follow that the opposite relationship would exist for at least one of the other two forms. This follows from the fact that, pooling the three forms, each drawing was paired with each statement one time. For example, if in one of the three forms the more muscular figures were more often paired with the symptom statement, "He is worried about how manly he is," it would necessarily follow that for another form the less muscular figures, rather than the more muscular ones, would be paired with this statement. Hence, if a drawing characteristic was reported as a correlate on the basis of a true relationship for one form, it would not be reported for one of the others. Table III shows these data. The three forms were found to be highly similar as to the drawing characteristics listed most often for each symptom. It follows that the reports cannot have been based on true relationships.

An examination of the data of Table II indicates support of the hypothesis that the most commonly reported illusory correlates are drawing characteristics with highest strength associative connection to the symptom statements. For example, it seems likely that suspiciousness tends to call to mind the eye more often than other parts of the body, and problems concerning intelligence tend to call to mind the head. In order to provide more objective evidence on this, a questionnaire was constructed for measuring the associative strength between the problem area of each symptom statement and the parts of the body that are referred to in the various drawing characteristics.

The problem areas of the symptom statements were each summarized as follows: "manliness," "suspiciousness," "intelligence," "being fed and cared

Table III

Percentage of Subjects Reporting the Most Popular Illusory Correlate of Each Symptom Statement

Symptom and drawing characteristic	Experiment 1 Forms			Experiment 2 Testings			Experiment 3 $N = 44$	Experiment 5 $N = 41$	Experiment 4 $N = 42$
	A $N = 34$	B $N = 38$	C $N = 36$	First $N = 56$	Second $N = 56$	Third $N = 56$			
1. Worry about manliness Manly, muscular	74	79	75	71	73	77	91	85	45
2. Suspicious Eyes atypical	59	53	77	52	50	48	55	56	36
3. Worry about intelligence Head emphasized	50	47	77	41	48	46	33	56	19
4. Need to be fed and cared for Feminine or childlike	50	45	27	21	21	23	45	44	24
5. Impotence Manly, muscular	44	29	27	25	27	30	34	27	10
6. Say bad things Facial expression atypical	26	63	77	50	50	48	45	63	45

for," "sexual impotence," and "bad things being said about one's self." The parts of the body with which association was measured for each of these were: shoulders and muscles, hair, eyes, head, mouth, genital organs, and ears. The six problem areas and seven body parts yielded 42 pairs, for each of which an item was constructed in the following format:

> The tendency for SUSPICIOUSNESS to call to mind HEAD is
> a. very strong
> b. strong
> c. moderate
> d. slight
> e. very slight
> f. no tendency at all

The questionnaire was given to a group of 45 undergraduate students who had not participated in the other studies reported in this paper.

The six associative ratings from "a" to "f" were assigned values of 6 to 1, and a mean was computed for each item. Table IV reports the mean rated associative strength for the 42 pairs. For each of the six symptoms, the highest strength associate was compared with the second highest by means of a direct difference t-test. The difference was found to be significant ($p <$ .001) for the first five symptoms, but not for the sixth ($t = 1.28; p = .20$).

The relationship of illusory correlation to associative strength can be seen by comparing the naive observers' responses in Table II with the associative ratings of Table IV. Taking one body part at a time, one finds, for all seven body parts, agreement between the two measures as to the symptom with which the body part has the strongest relationship. For example, Table IV shows that "eyes" are a stronger associate to "suspiciousness" than to any other symptom, and Table II shows that drawing characteristics mentioning "eyes" were an illusory correlate of that same symptom more often than any other symptom.

The data of the two tables may also be compared from the opposite starting point. Taking one symptom at a time, one may determine which of the seven body parts has the strongest relationship to it. Using this comparison, the agreement was again impressive but not perfect. For four of the six symptoms (numbers 1, 2, 3, and 5) the body part which was the strongest associate of the symptom was also the one most commonly reported in the drawing characteristics which were their illusory correlates. It is of interest to note that, for almost all of these comparisons, the correlates reported by the clinical psychologists were even more frequently the highest strength associate than was the case for the naive observers.

This finding that associative connection produces illusory correlation is congruent with the similar finding of the earlier laboratory studies that used only pairs of words as stimuli. The present results do not show that associative connection is the only source of illusory correlation in the DAP, but they do indicate that it is a major source.

Table IV

Mean Rated Associative Connection Between Problem Areas and Body Parts

Body part	Manliness	Suspiciousness	Intelligence	Fed and cared for	Impotence	Say bad things
Shoulders and muscles	4.8	1.3	1.7	1.8	1.8	1.3
Hair	2.4	1.2	1.3	1.6	1.5	1.5
Eyes	2.0	3.8	2.5	1.5	1.2	1.9
Head	2.3	1.8	4.3	1.6	1.5	1.8
Mouth	2.0	1.9	2.1	3.9	1.5	3.2
Genital organs	4.2	1.3	1.2	1.5	5.4	1.6
Ears	1.3	2.5	1.4	1.2	1.0	2.9

Experiment 2 — The Effects of Repeated Testing

The Ss in Experiment 1 had much less opportunity to observe the DAP protocols and the accompanying symptoms than do clinicians who interpret the DAP in clinical practice. One might wonder whether the experimental Ss would continue to show these same errors if given repeated opportunity to view the stimulus materials. Experiment 2 was designed to investigate this. Naive observers were given repeated experience with one of the three forms of the task used in Experiment 1.

Procedure. The Ss ($N = 56$) were shown the drawings and the symptom statements, followed by a questionnaire, at each of three sessions on consecutive days. The experimental procedure was substantially the same as in Experiment 1. The instructions on the first session were identical to those of Experiment 1, but on the second and third days they were shortened by eliminating the introductory material. Form A of the task was used on all three occasions.

Results. The responses at all three sessions were substantially the same as those in Experiment 1, and there was little change with repeated testings. At all three testings, the most frequently reported drawing characteristic for each of the six symptoms was the same as that of Experiment 1. Table III shows the drawing characteristic most often reported for each of the six symptoms and the percentage of Ss who reported it. As seen in Table III, these percentages remained highly stable across the three testings. A Cochran's Q analysis was used to determine whether any of the changes in percentage were significant. None approached the 5% level. From this we conclude that with stimulus materials of this type, repeated exposure does not reduce errors of illusory correlation.

Experiment 3 — The Effects of Guessing

The observers in Experiments 1 and 2 showed massive illusory correlation that appeared to be produced, in large part, by associative connection between the symptom statements and certain drawing characteristics. This suggests the possibility that the observers' illusory correlates may correspond to their prior expectations as to which stimuli are correlated in their occurrence. Many high strength associates are names of objects that tend to co-occur in everyone's daily experiences, for example, butter-bread and table-chair. The observers might be extending this principle to the DAP so that they expect symptoms and drawing characteristics that have an associative connection to be correlated in their occurrence. Experiment 3 was designed to test this possibility by asking Ss to guess the kinds of drawings made by men with each problem.

Procedure. The Ss ($N = 44$) were told about the DAP in the same manner as Ss in Experiment 1, but they were not shown any stimulus materials. They were then given the following instructions:

> Now we want to see what you can guess about this test. We have gathered a group of drawings by men with various emotional problems. In each case, we asked the patient to draw a picture of a man.

The Ss were then given a questionnaire which listed an item in the following format for each of the six symptom statements.

He is worried about how manly he is.

> The pictures drawn by such men would more often be characterized by
> 1. ....
> 2. ....
> 3. ....

Results. The responses were found to resemble closely those of the naive observers in Experiments 1 and 2. The most frequently guessed drawing characteristic for each of the six symptoms was the same as the one most frequently reported by Ss of those two studies. Table III lists the percentage of Ss who guessed each of these six relationships.

The similarity of the guesses to the reports of illusory correlates in the first two studies indicates that the illusory correlates corresponded to the observers' expectations. This also leads one to suspect that the similar observations by practicing psychodiagnosticians may also be based on the same prior expectations.

Experiment 4 — The Effects of True Correlations Opposing the Illusory Ones

The finding of Experiment 3 that the blind guesses of naive Ss closely resemble their observational reports might lead one to speculate that the illusory correlates reported by Ss in Experiments 1 and 2 might be attributable to their failing to perceive the stimulus materials. This might result either through lack of motivation to attend to the task or insufficient opportunity to do so in the time allotted. Actually, Ss seemed to be interested in the material and highly motivated to discover the relationships between the symptoms and the drawings. Also, no one complained about lack of time for determining the correct answers. Nevertheless, it seemed necessary to attempt to rule out these interpretations by means of appropriate experiments. The first such study was Experiment 4.

In Experiment 4, the task materials of Experiments 1 and 2 were altered so as to introduce true correlations between certain symptom statements and drawing characteristics. The expectation was that if Ss were truly attending to the task, their responses to these altered materials would differ from the responses made in Experiments 1 and 2.

Procedure. The same drawings and symptom statements were used as in Experiments 1 and 2, but the pattern of assignment of the symptom statements to the various drawings was altered. They were assigned so that, for each of five symptoms, there was a strong negative correlation between the occurrence of the symptom statement and one drawing characteristic which had often been reported as occurring with it in the earlier studies. For example, in both studies it was reported that the symptom statement of worry about intelligence was most often accompanied by a drawing of a figure with a head that was either large or emphasized in some other way. Therefore, in the present study the 15 presentations of the statement "He is worried about how intelligent he is" were not paired with any of the figures with large heads, but were instead paired only with the smallest heads. A similar negative correlation was built in between four other symptom statements and drawing characteristics. These symptoms and drawing characteristics are listed in Table V. Note that the categories of drawing characteristics are more narrowly defined than the categories used in Tables II and III. The categories were chosen so that the true negative relationships could be built in unambiguously. For example, the category "large eyes" was used instead of "atypical eyes" which included not only large eyes, but also eyes that were staring, slanted, beady, etc.

Table V

Percentage of Subjects Who Reported Each of Five Illusory Correlates
in Experiment 1 and Experiment 4

Symptom and drawing characteristic*	Experiment 1 (N = 108)	Experiment 4 (N = 38)	P
1. Worry about manliness Manly, muscular	76	50	.01
2. Suspicious Large or elaborate eyes	28	8	.02
3. Worry about intelligence Large heads	44	16	.01
4. Need to be fed and cared for Childlike figures	25	3	.01
5. Impotence Manly, muscular	31	21	ns
Mean percentage	41	20	

*Note that the drawing characteristics are more narrowly defined for Symptoms
2, 3, and 4 than in Table III.

This task was presented to the Ss (N = 38) in the same manner as in
Experiment 1. The prediction was that Ss would respond to these true
negative correlations by reducing the number of erroneous reports of the
contrary positive illusory correlates.

Results. The responses were tabulated in the same manner as in the previous
studies. Table V lists the percentage of Ss who reported observing the five
illusory positive correlates. In each case, the illusory correlate is in the
direction opposite to that which is objectively present. As seen in Table V,
these five illusory correlates were reported only about half as often as in
Experiment 1. Chi-square analysis indicated that the reduction in frequency
of report was significant for four of the five.

It is clear, therefore, that Ss were attending to the materials much of the
time and that the illusory correlation found in Experiments 1 and 2 cannot
be attributed solely to Ss failing to attend. Nevertheless, the data of Table V
reveal that the illusory correlates show surprisingly strong survival in the face
of true contrary correlates. Is this residual illusory correlation attributable to
the strength of the error, or might it instead by attributable to insufficient
time or low motivation of some of the Ss? The next study, Experiment 5, was
designed to test these possibilities more directly.

Experiment 5 — The Effects of Enhanced Motivation

The Ss (N = 41) in Experiment 5 were tested under circumstances designed to maximize both their motivation to observe accurately and their opportunity to do so. The task materials were Form A from Experiment 1, in which there was no true correlation between symptom statements and drawing characteristics. As in Experiments 1, 2, and 4, Ss were told that their task was to observe what kinds of drawings were made by men with each kind of problem. However, a prize of $20 was offered for the S who was most accurate in his observations. Also, unlike the earlier studies, Ss were tested individually and were permitted to look at each drawing and its symptom statements as long as they wished. However, they were not permitted to look at more than one drawing at a time and were required to look at them in a prearranged random order. They were not permitted to return to a picture after they had once put it down.

In order to make the contest more realistic, the questionnaire was modified to request an additional bit of information. The Ss were asked to list, for each drawing characteristic that they reported as drawn by patients with a given symptom, the percentage of such patients who showed it. However, these latter data were not analyzed.

Results. Surprisingly, the observational reports made under these conditions were quite similar to those of Experiments 1, 2, and 3. For each of the six symptoms, the drawing characteristic most often listed as its correlate was the same as in those studies. Table III shows the percentage of Ss who reported each of these correlates. Chi-square analysis indicated that none of the percentages was significantly different from those of Experiment 1.

Since the illusory correlation was not reduced by the prospect of a $20 prize for accuracy of observation combined with unlimited viewing time, one may conclude that it is not attributable either to lack of motivation or lack of time to view the stimulus materials.

Experiment 6 — The Effects of Enhanced Motivation with Unlimited Viewing Opportunities

The findings of Experiment 5 led to the question of what are the conditions of observation that might reduce the incidence of report of these illusory correlates. In Experiment 6, Ss were tested under conditions designed to facilitate greatly their accuracy so that they might discover that the illusory correlates were unwarranted.

The task materials used were again Form A and the same questionnaire as in Experiment 5. The Ss were given the questionnaire together with the stack of cards, as well as scratch paper, a ruler, and a pencil. Again, a $20 prize was offered to the S who was most accurate. Unlike Experiment 5, Ss were allowed to shuffle the cards, rearrange them, compare groups of cards, and return to any card as often as they wished. Thus Ss could, if they wished, sort the cards with a given symptom into one pile and those with a second symptom into another pile, spread out the two piles of pictures and compare them. However, not all Ss went to this much effort. Table III shows the percentage of Ss who reported each of the illusory correlates that, in the previous studies, had been most often reported for each of the six symptoms.

As seen in Table III, there was a drop from Experiment 1 in the percentage of Ss reporting these six illusory correlates. The drop was significant ($p < .05$) for Symptoms 1, 2, 3, and 5, but it fell short of significance for the other two. The mean of the six percentages was 52% in Experiment 1 and 30% in the present study.

Although the frequency of report of these illusory correlates dropped under these conditions, the most striking aspect of the findings is the resistance of the error to the influence of reality.

Experiment 7 — Consensual Pseudovalidation in Psychodiagnostic Observation

The conditions of observation in these laboratory studies differed from that of the practicing psychodiagnostician. The observers in these studies, unlike psychodiagnosticians in clinical practice, were not allowed to communicate with one another. Clinicians usually discuss their observations with one another and, on finding agreement, are reassured of their accuracy. Our findings indicate, however, that agreement may often reflect shared error rather than shared accuracy. One might describe such agreement as "consensual pseudovalidation." The observers would be strengthened in their conviction that the correlations are valid, despite the fact that the correlations are illusory.

Experiment 7 was a study of the enhancement of illusory correlation by consensual pseudovalidation. This enhancement of illusory correlation was studied both in terms of increased frequency of report of popular illusory correlates, and of increased confidence in the accuracy of the erroneous observations.

The task materials were identical to those of Form A, Experiment 1. After all of the Ss ($N = 43$) had seen all 45 pictures, they were given a questionnaire like that described above for Experiment 1, with the addition of a confidence rating for the accuracy of each report of a drawing characteristic for a symptom.

After the 43 Ss had observed the 45 cards and filled out the questionnaire, they were divided into five discussion groups and told to compare their responses. They were instructed to discuss one symptom statement at a time, to take turns reading the drawing characteristics that each member had recorded as correlates of that symptom, to discuss the extent to which they agreed or did not agree with one another, and to attempt to arrive at a consensus as to the true correlate of the symptom. They were not allowed, however, to alter their written protocols.

The Ss returned for a second testing the next day. At this session, the Ss were shown the same task materials as at their first testing, and they were given the same questionnaire. However, they did not discuss their observations after recording.

Questionnaires from the two testings were compared as to the frequency of report of the three most popular illusory correlates. These three correlates, all of which correspond to high strength verbal associative connection, were (1) broad shoulders, muscular or manly – for worry about manliness, (2) head, large or emphasized – for worry about intelligence, and (3) atypical eyes – for suspiciousness. The frequency of report of these three illusory correlates was found to increase between the first and second testings (t = 2.16, $p < .05$), as shown by a direct difference t-test. The Ss' ratings of their confidence in their observations also increased from the first to the second testing ($t = 4.46, p < .005$).

The increase in frequency of report of associatively based illusory correlates differs from results of Experiment 2 in which repeated observation was investigated without provision for discussion of observations. The observers in Experiment 2 did not change the frequency of report of the popular illusory correlates with repeated testings. These results indicate that opportunity to discuss observations of clinical materials strengthens the report of the illusory correlate.

Illusory Correlation as an Obstacle to the Use of Valid Psychodiagnostic Signs

Our studies on illusory correlation in the observation of DAP signs are open to one logically possible alternative interpretation. Some clinicians might claim that, despite the massive negative experimental evidence, the signs that the naive Ss reported as illusory correlates are all valid in real life. The naive observers may have guessed this truth and, as a result, believed that they observed the same signs to be valid in the contrived task materials of the experiments. This alternative interpretation is a logically possible one, even if highly unlikely. The next group of studies were designed to demonstrate illusory correlation in observation of psychodiagnostic signs for which this alternative interpretation is clearly unsupportable. These were studies of the report of associatively based, illusory correlates of a symptom in a psychodiagnostic test in which there are valid test signs for the symptom, but the valid test signs and symptom lack a strong verbal associative connection.

The hypothesis was that both practicing clinicians and naive observers would overlook the valid test signs and would instead report observing signs that are objectively invalid, but have a strong verbal associative connection to the symptom.

These studies required a test which research has demonstrated to have valid signs for some symptom, but for which clinicians prefer invalid signs. The Rorschach Test was chosen because it appears to fulfill these criteria in content analysis for male homosexuality. Wheeler (1949) offered 20 Rorschach content signs of male homosexuality. Many clinicians report having observed some of these signs to be valid in their own clinical experience, but research evidence strongly supports two of the signs that are not popular among clinicians. Three separate sets of investigators (Davids, Joelson, & McArthur, 1956; Hooker, 1958; Wheeler, 1949) have reported statistically interpretable evidence on the validity of all 20 Wheeler-Rorschach signs, and these studies show some agreement.

Wheeler Signs 7 and 8 were both found to distinguish homosexual from heterosexual groups at the 5% level (using a one-tailed test) by two of the three studies (Sign 7 by Wheeler and by Davids *et al.*; Sign 8 by Davids *et al.* and by Hooker). Wheeler Sign 7 is a response on Card IV of "human or animal — contorted, monstrous, or threatening," and Wheeler Sign 8 is a response on Card V, W or Center detail, of a "human, or humanized animal." Signs 10, 17, 19, and 20 were each found to distinguish the groups in one study but were tested and not found valid in the other two studies. A finding by chance alone, of a significant difference for one or two signs out of 20 is not unexpected in a study. Therefore, for purposes of the present paper, only Signs 7 and 8 will be considered clinically valid signs. A fourth study (Reitzell, 1949) tends to support this conclusion. She reported Signs 7, 8, and 16 as the most discriminating of the 20 Wheeler signs. (Unfortunately, she reported her data in a form not amenable to statistical analyses.)

We performed a series of studies that were somewhat analogous in design to those reported above for the Draw-A-Person Test.

Experiment 1 — Survey of Observations by Psychodiagnosticians in Clinical Practice

First, we surveyed a group of psychodiagnosticians as to the kinds of content that they have observed clinically in the Rorschach responses of male homosexuals. Our hypothesis was that the frequency of report of signs by the practicing psychodiagnosticians would have little relationship to the objective clinical validity of the signs as indicated by research evidence, but would instead be predictable by strength of verbal associative connection of the signs to the symptom of male homosexuality. This prediction was confirmed. None of the clinicians who responded to the survey ($N = 32$) reported observing either Sign 7 or Sign 8, which were the two valid signs, as a correlate of male homosexuality. They most frequently reported observing Wheeler Sign 16 (human or animal anal content) — 40%, Sign 20 (feminine clothing) — 38%, Sign 19 (male or female genitalia) — 38%, Sign 4 (humans with sex confused) — 28%, and Sign 5 (humans with sex uncertain) — 16%.

The hypothesis that popularity of signs was based on verbal associative connection was tested by means of ratings on strength of verbal associative connection between homosexuality and each of the five popular invalid signs and to each of the two unpopular valid signs. The ratings were obtained from college students using a rating scale in the format described above for the DAP.

The predictions were confirmed. All five of the popular invalid signs were found to have a significantly stronger associative connection to male homosexuality than either of the two unpopular clinically valid signs.

Experiment 2 — Illusory Correlation in the Absence of Valid Correlations

A series of laboratory studies were designed to determine whether naive observers, when presented with contrived statements of patients' symptoms and their Rorschach responses, would make the same errors of observation that the psychodiagnosticians appear to have made in their clinical practice. Such a demonstration would lend strong additional support to the contention that the clinicians' reports reflected illusory correlation based on associative connection.

The first experiment was designed to determine if the invalid signs that were found to be popular with the clinicians would also be reported by naive observers viewing materials contrived so that no true correlation was present between any category of percepts and the symptom of male homosexuality.

Clinical materials were fabricated in much the same manner as described above for the DAP. The materials consisted of 30 Rorschach cards, on each of which one percept (or response) was indicated. The 30 percepts were chosen so that they fell into five categories, namely: one popular invalid sign (either Sign 16, 20, 19, 4, or 5), the two popular valid signs (Signs 7 and 8), and two filler categories of percepts. The five popular invalid signs required five conditions in all. Each percept was paired with two statements of the emotional problems of the patient who was alleged to have given the percept. Percepts were indicated by circling an area of the card and pasting in a corner a typed statement of the response. For example, for one of the 30 Rorschach responses, the center area of Card V (Beck's area D-7) was circled and labeled "Bugs Bunny." In a corner of the card the following statement appeared:

The man who said this

1. has sexual feelings toward other men.
2. feels sad and depressed much of the time.

The statements of emotional problems or symptoms on the cards were drawn from a pool of four such statements, namely:

1. He has sexual feelings toward other men.
2. He believes other people are plotting against him.
3. He feels sad and depressed much of the time.
4. He has strong feelings of inferiority.

The statements of symptoms and Rorschach percepts were paired on the 30 cards so that each symptom occurred equally often with each category of percept.

Each S viewed each of the 30 cards for 60 seconds. He was then given a questionnaire which presented items in the following format.

Some of the things in the ink blots were seen by men who have the following problem:

He has sexual feelings toward other men

Did you notice any general kind of thing that was seen most often by men with this problem? Yes _____ No _____ . If your answer is yes, name that kind of thing, and give one example of that kind of thing.
Kind of thing _____
Example _____

Results. Only 11% of the Ss indicated that they had not noticed any kind of percept that was seen most often by men with this problem. In each condition, the Ss reported, as predicted, that they observed the hypothesized illusory correlate as accompanying homosexual problems more often than any other category of percept. Altogether, 44% of the observers reported associatively based illusory correlates, that is, the clinically popular invalid signs. The clinically valid signs were reported as a correlate of homosexuality by an average of only 8% of the observers, despite the equivalency of its objective occurrence to that of the associatively based percepts. These findings mean that the erroneous report of popular invalid Rorschach signs of male homosexuality were reproduced in the laboratory as associatively based illusory correlates.

Experiment 3 — Illusory Correlation in the Presence of Valid Correlations

In this study, the covariations of symptom with test signs more closely approximated those of the real life clinical situation. Naive observers were tested in a series of conditions in which the clinically valid signs had a contrived validity in the experimental task materials. The designs in these conditions were identical to those of the immediately previous study except that the clinically valid Wheeler Signs 7 and 8 were paired with the symptom statement of homosexuality more often than with the other symptoms.

Three degrees of contrived validity were used: one in which the symptom of homosexuality was stated with two-thirds of the percepts of each of the two valid signs, one in which it was stated with five-sixths of them, and one in which it was stated with all of them. Each of the four symptom statements accompanied 50% of each of the other categories of percepts.

Results. The associatively based illusory correlates proved to be impervious to the influence of competing valid correlations. The clinically popular invalid sign was the most frequently reported correlate of the symptom statement for all three degrees of contrived validity of the valid correlates. The clinically popular invalid signs were reported as a correlate of homosexuality by an average of 47% of the observers, almost exactly the same percentage as in the conditions in which no valid correlates were built into the task. Altogether, the two valid signs were reported only an average of 15% apiece.

Experiment 4 — Accuracy of Report in the Absence of Invalid Popular Signs

The findings of the above study might lead one to wonder if the infrequent detection of valid signs on these tasks is truly due to the distracting influence of illusory correlates, or if, instead, the valid signs are difficult to discover, regardless of the presence or absence of associatively based illusory correlates. Experiment 4 was designed to obtain evidence on this question. The stimulus materials differed only slightly from those of the two conditions of the previous study in which the symptom statement of homosexuality accompanied five-sixths of the percepts of the two clinically valid signs (Signs 7 & 8) and accompanied only 50% of each of the other categories of percepts. The only change from the previous study was that there was no popular invalid sign (illusory correlate) presented, but an extra filler category of percepts was substituted for it.

Results. In these conditions, the two clinically valid signs were the most frequently reported categories of percepts, about double the percentage reported in the conditions in which illusory correlates were present. (One valid sign was reported by 27% of the observers and the other by 38%.) These results demonstrated that the task of observing correlates is not so intrinsically difficult that an observer cannot respond to reality. One must instead conclude that in Experiments 1, 2, and 3 the presence of illusory correlates reduced accuracy of observation.

Discussion

The findings of all these studies are markedly consistent. They demonstrate that when naive observers are shown test responses together with statements of the symptoms of the alleged patients who made the responses, the observers show marked agreement in erroneously reporting the same kinds of test responses as correlates of the symptoms. The test responses that they erroneously report as correlates are those that have strong verbal associative connections to the symptoms. The observers persist in reporting these illusory correlates, both under repeated exposure to the stimulus materials and under conditions designed to maximize motivation and opportunity to observe accurately. They report the illusory correlates even in the presence of competing valid correlates of the symptoms. These associatively based illusory correlates are almost completely congruent with the kinds of test responses that practicing psychodiagnosticians most often erroneously report as correlates of the same symptoms. This striking congruence indicates that many clinical observations have their genesis in illusory correlation arising from associative connection. When the task provided no associatively based stimuli that could serve as illusory correlates, accuracy of observation of valid correlates rose. This indicates that the report of illusory correlates cannot be interpreted as simply a reliance on an expected relationship in an impossibly difficult task. Further evidence on this point is the finding that the offer of a $20 prize for accuracy, and unlimited viewing time did not eliminate illusory correlation.

The conditions of observation in these laboratory studies appear more suitable for accurate observation than the conditions of conventional clinical practice. In the laboratory studies, Ss observed the various symptom statements and drawings within a short time of one another. In clinical practice, the time to accumulate observations of patients with the same symptoms is often a period of months, or even years, which should facilitate selective forgetting. In these laboratory studies, the number of symptoms for each patient was limited to two and were unambiguously stated, while in clinical practice, there are usually so many that the clinician has difficulty deciding which are the most important.

Consensual pseudovalidation enhanced frequency of report of the illusory correlates in Experiment 7 on the DAP despite the fact that the observers communicated on only one brief occasion during the experimental sessions. Psychodiagnosticians, in clinical practice, have more frequent access to the observations of their colleagues. They are repeatedly reassured as to the accuracy of their observations by their fellow workers, who themselves observe the same illusory correlates. Such consensual validation, especially among experts, is usually regarded as evidence of accuracy.

The studies reviewed here indicate that illusory correlation in observations by clinicians do not reflect personal defects of the clinicians, but instead, are inherent in the clinicians' task. The errors are ones to which most, or perhaps all, people are prone. By analogy, if the practitioners of some profession had as their task the estimation of the length of lines, these practitioners surely would not be criticized if most of them were subject to the Muller-Lyer illusion.

How might one hope to obtain accurate psychodiagnostic observation? One partial solution might be special training. Graduate students in clinical psychology could be asked to serve as observers in a task like those used in the present studies, and could be shown the nature of their own illusory correlates. They would then perhaps have a keener awareness of the difficulties of making such observations, and would be less likely to make errors of illusory correlation in future clinical practice. Hopefully, such training would also make students more receptive to relevant research evidence.

Training in the dangers of illusory correlation would not, however, solve the more fundamental problem of how to make accurate statements about patients on the basis of test performance. The difficulty is that the psychodiagnostician's task of information processing often exceeds the capacity of the human intellect. The ultimate solution, as suggested by Meehl (1960) and other workers, will probably be at least a partial replacement of subjective clinical psychodiagnostic methods by the method of objective cookbook formulae, derived actuarially.

Not all patients, however, can be conveniently cast into an actuarial formula. There will probably always be some patients whom the psycho-diagnostician recognizes as atypical from the Ss in the standardization samples used for deriving the available actuarial formulae. The psychodiag-nostician must, if he is to make accurate statements about such patients, maintain an awareness of the dangers of illusory correlation.

References

Bastian, J. Associative factors in verbal transfer. *Journal of Experimental Psychology*, 1961, **62**, 70-79.

Beck, S. *Rorschach's test.* Vol. I. *Basic processes.* (3rd ed.) New York: Grune & Stratton, 1961.

Chapman, L. J. A search for lunacy. *Journal of Nervous and Mental Disease*, 1961, **132**, 171-74.

Chapman, L. J. Illusory correlation in observational report. *Journal of Verbal Learning and Verbal Behavior*, 1967, **6**, 151-55.

Chapman, L. J. & Chapman, J. P. The genesis of popular but erroneous psychodiagnostic observations. *Journal of Abnormal Psychology*, 1967, **72**, 193-204.

Chapman, L. J. & Chapman, J. P. Illusory correlation as an obstacle to the use of valid psychodiagnostic signs. *Journal of Abnormal Psychology*, in press.

Davids, A., Joelson, M., & McArthur, C. Rorschach and TAT indices of homosexuality in overt homosexuals, neurotics, and normal males. *Journal of Abnormal and Social Psychology*, 1956, **53**, 161-72.

Eron, L. D. A normative study of the Thematic Apperception Test. *Psychological Monographs*, 1950, **64** (Whole No. 315).

Fisher, S. & Fisher, R. Test of certain assumptions regarding figure drawing analysis. *Journal of Abnormal and Social Psychology*, 1950, **45**, 727-32.

Frazer, J. G. *The golden bough.* Part I. *The magic art.* New York: MacMillan, 1935.

Freud, S. *The basic writings of . . . Totem and taboo.* New York: Modern Library, 1938.

Goldberg, L. R. Simple models or simple processes? Some research on clinical judgments. *American Psychologist*, 1968, **23**, 483-96.

Griffith, A. V. & Peyman, P. A. R. Eye-ear emphasis in the DAP as indicating ideas of reference. *Journal of Consulting Psychology*, 1959, **23**, 560.

Haagen, C. H. Synonymity, vividness, familiarity, and association value ratings of 400 pairs of common adjectives. *Journal of Psychology*, 1949, **27**, 453-63.

Hammer, E. F. & Piotrowski, Z. A. Hostility as a factor in the clinician's personality as it affects his interpretation of projective drawings (H-T-P). *Journal of Projective Techniques*, 1953, **17**, 210-16.

Holzberg, J. D. & Wexler, M. The validity of human form drawings as a measure of personality deviation. *Journal of Projective Techniques*, 1950, 14, 343-61.

Hooker, E. Male homosexuality in the Rorschach. *Journal of Projective Techniques*, 1958, 22, 33-54.

Little, K. B. & Shneidman, E. S. Congruencies among interpretations of psychological test and anamnestic data. *Psychological Monographs*, 1959, 73 (6, Whole No. 476).

Machover, K. *Personality projection in the drawing of the human figure.* Springfield, Ill.: (Charles C.) Thomas, 1949.

Masling, J. M. The influence of situational and interpersonal variables in projective testing. *Psychological Bulletin*, 1960, 57, 65-85.

Meehl, P. E. The cognitive activity of the clinician. *American Psychologist*, 1960, 15, 19-27.

Radford, E. & Radford, M. A. *Encyclopedia of superstitions.* New York: Philosophical Library, 1949.

Ravitz, L. J. Electrocyclic phenomena and emotional states. *Journal of Clinical and Experimental Psychopathology*, 1952, 13, 69-106.

Ravitz, L. J. Electrodynamic field theory in psychiatry. *Southern Medical Journal*, 1953, 46, 650-60.

Ravitz, L. J. Comparative clinical and electrocyclic observations on twin brothers concordant as to schizophrenia. *Journal of Nervous and Mental Disease*, 1955, 121, 72-87.

Reitzell, J. M. A comparative study of hysterics, homosexuals and alcoholics using content analysis of Rorschach responses. *Rorschach Research Exchange*, 1949, 13, 127-41.

Reznikoff, M. & Nicholas, A. L. An evaluation of human figure drawing indicators of paranoid pathology. *Journal of Consulting Psychology*, 1958, 22, 395-97.

Ribler, R. I. Diagnostic prediction from emphasis on the eye and the ear in human figure drawings. *Journal of Consulting Psychology*, 1957, 21, 223-25.

Roback, H. B. Human figure drawings: Their utility in the clinical psychologist's armamentarium for personality assessment. *Psychological Bulletin*, 1968, 70, 1-19.

Rotter, J. B. Thematic Apperception Tests: Suggestions for administration and interpretation. *Journal of Personality*, 1946, 15, 70-92.

Sundberg, N. D. The practice of psychological testing in clinical services in the United States. *American Psychologist*, 1961, 16, 79-83.

Swensen, C. H. Empirical evaluations of human figure drawings. *Psychological Bulletin*, 1957, 54, 431-66.

Swensen, C. H. Empirical evaluations of human figure drawings: 1957-1966. *Psychological Bulletin*, 1968, 70, 20-44.

Temkin, O. *The falling sickness.* Baltimore: Johns Hopkins Press, 1945.

Thorndike, E. L. A constant error in psychological ratings. *Journal of Applied Psychology*, 1920, 4, 25-29.

Underwood, B. J. & Goad, D. Studies of distributed practice: I. The influence of intra-list similarity in serial learning. *Journal of Experimental Psychology*, 1951, 42, 125-34.

Wheeler, W. M. An analysis of Rorschach indices of male homosexuality. *Rorschach Research Exchange*, 1949, 13, 97-126.

Zubin, J., Eron, L. D. & Schumer, F. *An experimental approach to projective techniques.* New York: Wiley, 1965.

Chapter 4

Psychological Intervention in a Community Crisis [1]

Sidney E. Cleveland

The Diffident Psychologist

A criticism frequently leveled at today's average citizen is his failure to become involved in meeting the problems posed by his neighborhood, his community, and his society. Until recently, psychologists have been equally remiss in failing to become involved in the major social movements confronting them. Psychologists traditionally have preferred the relative solitude of the scientific laboratory and the academic halls to the clamor of the street, the din of the marketplace, and the blare of the ghetto. All too often in the recent past, psychologists have shunned the responsibility of applying their scientific findings and hypotheses to the practical problems of their communities. Psychologists in academic settings have preferred to remain in the classroom or, if venturing into the arena of behavioral problems, to stray no further from the campus than the university counseling center. Psychologists in private practice have generally been no bolder and have preferred the comfort of their office to the squalor of the street below. Sanford (1958) commented on the reluctance of psychologists to abandon their scientific humility and assume some visibility in the practical affairs of living. Speaking at that time of the embarrassment displayed by psychologists when faced with public exposure, he noted:

> . . .psychologists are possessed of more diffidence than is good for them. As a breed we instinctively dodge visibility. We do not, except under great pressure . . ., speak our minds on issues of general interest. We have a passion for dodging the spotlight of public responsibility and a genius for avoiding direct and unqualified statements. (p. 81)

[1] Portions of this chapter are adapted from papers prepared by Dr. Robert L. Bell, Dr. Philip G. Hanson, Dr. Walter E. O'Connell, and the present author, comprising a symposium entitled "Innovations in Police Techniques: Community Service and Community Relations," presented at the 76th Annual Convention of the American Psychological Association, San Francisco, California, August 30-September 3, 1968. I am indebted to Drs. Bell, Hanson, and O'Connell for their contributions to this chapter.

Sanford went on to encourage his fellow psychologists to become directly involved in the broad practical problems presented by the social movements of the time:

> If the culture moves ahead into an era of scientific humanism – and it seems a good guess that it will – it will look more and more to the psychologist for guidance and facilitation. If the psychologist can maintain his identity, if he can find ways to combine humanistic values with the morality of science, then there is enormous challenge and opportunity and responsibility ahead. (p. 85)

The ensuing 10 years have seen psychology grasp the challenge and responsibility contained in Sanford's remarks. In increasing numbers, psychologists have entered the public arena to grapple with messy and untidy problems. Problems of the ghetto, the selection, training, and evaluation of Peace Corps candidates for service around the world, and the involvement of psychologists in community health projects serve as testimonials to the surge of psychology into the real problems of living.

Foremost among these problems is that of our urban crisis, most often expressed in terms of the rising antagonism between the police and residents of the urban ghettos. Most of our communities are undergoing a period of social change. Many traditional social attitudes, social groupings, and customs are rapidly being altered. New social and political groups are evolving to challenge the authority and practices of established interests. The sense of urgency and insistence accompanying demands for change gives rise to tension within the community, distrust, unsettling rumors, and sometimes physical confrontations. Most often it is the city police force that is thrust directly into the fray and serves as the primary mediator for urban tension. Inevitably, charges of police brutality and misbehavior, alleged or real, arise to complicate a difficult situation. The relationship between police and community becomes a focal point for friction and the detonation device leading to violent explosions. The *President's Riot Commission Report*, by the National Advisory Commission on Civil Disorders has found that "almost invariably the incident that ignites disorder arises from police action" (1968, p. 206). Hostility toward the police is often so intense that even routine and legal police procedures antagonize ordinarily law-abiding ghetto residents. Since, for many members of minority groups, the police symbolize all that is hated and feared in white society, the police officer unfortunately receives hostility which actually has very little to do with him (i.e., hostility generated by intolerable social conditions such as inadequate housing and under-employment). Actual police misconduct, as documented by four national commissions, further intensifies hostility toward the police (Wickersham Commission, 1931; President's Commission, 1947; State Advisory Committees, 1961; U. S. Riot Commission, 1968).

Psychologists have shown a willingness to assist in the resolution of this enormously complex and emotionally supercharged situation. Following disturbances in Boston, a police-community relations program was initiated, sponsored by the Boston University Training Center in Youth Development (Saal, 1967). The Newark riot was followed by a program of team building between police and ghetto residents (Saal, 1967). Bard and Berkowitz (1967) have reported on an innovative program of family crisis intervention, using specially trained police teams as a community mental health resource. Mills (1968) has described an elaborate psychological screening program developed to assist in the selection of mature and psychologically balanced police recruits for the Cincinnati police force.

The Houston Cooperative Crime Prevention Project

Background to the Problem

Probably the most intensive police-community relations program, one involving the largest number of officers and community members, is the Houston program initiated in October 1967. As was the case with most of these crisis oriented community programs, the doctor was called only after the patient had exhibited alarming symptoms. In Houston, a program to alleviate police-community tensions was initiated only after violence had erupted.

Prior to the outbreak of actual violence in Houston, there were many indications of increasingly tense race relations. In January of 1966, a confidential federal survey listed Houston as one of 21 United States cities where black unrest represented a ready potential for racial explosion (Adams, 1967). As has been the case in many of the large cities which have had direct physical confrontations between the police and the Negro community, Houston had numerous incidents which suggested that the relationship between Negroes and the police was particularly strained. The *President's Riot Commission Report*, recorded at least 10 separate incidents prior to the outbreak of actual violence. Nevertheless, the official representatives of the people of Houston frequently pointed with apparent pride at the "progress" in race relations in the city and maintained that, because of this progress, Houston had no problems of any significance in the racial sphere. Just as the city seemed the most confident of its racial harmony, a disturbance occurred at Texas Southern University, a predominantly Negro institution located in Houston. Four hours of gunfire between students at Texas Southern University and the Houston Police Department occurred on May 16-17, 1967. There are many versions of what took place at TSU, but two opposing views seem to dominate the speculations concerning what actually happened. One version (Helmer, 1967) is described as follows:

> Avenging a comrade slain by one of their own stray bullets, six hundred maddened, cursing cossacks of the Houston Police Department riddled the

> dormitories of Texas Southern University with six thousand shots, stormed
> in with clubs and gun butts swinging, and then methodically destroyed the
> student's personal property and living quarters. (p. 1)

An opposing version (Helmer, 1967) "relates the policemen's ordeal, their hours of patience, their futile efforts to negotiate a truce, their abuse by bullets and profanity, their remarkable restraint in quelling a dangerous riot without injury to a single student." (p. 1)

Obviously what happened at TSU has been extremely difficult to reconstruct, and reality lies somewhere between these extremes. Press reports were inconsistent, sketchy, and provoked many still unanswered questions. Some observers contended that the disturbance constituted a police riot or at least an overreaction by the police. Others maintained that the students were rioting and needed to be stopped by whatever methods the police deemed necessary.

Racial tensions increased after the TSU incident and many people became alarmed and feared another Watts or another Detroit. Subsequent action by the city government seemed to further intensify racial tensions. For example, five TSU students were indicted and charged with murder, despite the fact that there appeared to be little evidence that the officer who had been killed was hit by a bullet from the same caliber gun alleged to be used by students firing on the police. In fact, there is the possibility that, in the wild melee, the officer was struck by a ricocheting police bullet. However, there was a widespread belief in the Negro community that these students were selected as scapegoats for the city. Thus the gap between whites and blacks increased.

A study by Justice (1968), a psychologist and an assistant to the mayor on race relations, found that Negro antagonism toward the police had increased significantly over the pre-TSU riot period. Three surveys on attitudes toward the police had been completed prior to the TSU incident. A team of Negro interviewers studied attitudes of Negroes concerning jobs, wages, schools, housing, police, integration, effects of riots, and the use of violence; 1798 randomly selected Negro citizens from 22 Negro neighborhoods were interviewed. After the TSU incident, the study was repeated in the same neighborhoods to assess attitudinal changes. Results of these surveys indicated a significant rise (.01 level) in hostile feelings toward the police following the TSU incident. An example of the Justice study findings is contained in Table I, where the pre- and post-TSU riot reactions of the Negro community are presented in response to the question, "How do you think police treat Negroes in Houston?"

The results of this survey were influential in persuading the city administration that some type of educational or advisory program was needed to reduce existing tensions within the city. Originally the city advisors had in mind a lecture series on community relations to be presented to the police.

Table I

**Perceived Treatment of Negroes by Houston Police
Before and After TSU Incident**

Perceived Police Treatment	Black Community % Before TSU	Black Community % After TSU
Very good — fairly good	52	24
Fairly bad — very bad	37	67
Don't know	11	9

Dr. Melvin P. Sikes[2], then a clinical psychologist on the staff at the Houston VA Hospital, was asked to organize such a program. Similar programs conducted in other cities were studied, and while most of these comprised a lecture-discussion series, such a format was not felt to be promising in reducing tensions within the community. A lecture-discussion approach would not only leave the police unexposed to a direct expression of feelings and problems by the community, but would provide only minimal involvement on the part of officers. In addition, it was felt that the police would resent outside experts advising them on their problems in the community. More direct and active communication and exchange between community and officers was considered desirable. Accordingly, a decision was made to devise a program involving the entire Houston police force and as many community members as feasible, providing small group interaction between the officers and participating community. It seemed that a Human Relations Training Laboratory approach would be most appropriate, since such a format would permit the participants to express, exchange, and challenge mutual images and attitudes, as well as work together in seeking resolution of conflicts which arose in the group discussions.

Problems of Organization

This was a difficult program to initiate. Although there was very little active opposition to the setting up of a program, there was a pervasive feeling that no one really wanted to get involved in what appeared to be a controversial undertaking. The few community leaders who were aware of the possibility that a police-community relations program would be inaugurated

[2]Now at the University of Texas, Austin.

expressed fears that an open discussion of police-minority group problems would intensify rather than alleviate conflict. Others feared that the initiation of the program would be tantamount to admitting police misconduct and would undermine public confidence in the police. The administrators of the police department were also reluctant to become involved in the program, although they ultimately agreed to allow their men to participate.

The financing of the program had to be considered. Since the program was designed to include every member of the police department in small discussion groups meeting once weekly for six weeks, the cost for undertaking the program was quite high — much too high to be supported with funds from the current city budget. Although there are federal sources which might have provided at least partial support for a program of this nature, Houston is a relatively anti-federal Government city. Consequently, the idea of utilizing federal funds was rejected.

An appeal for funds was made to 40 top-level Houston businessmen. The Justice study findings on the effects of racial violence on Negro attitudes toward the police were used by the Mayor's office to demonstrate to these men the urgency of taking immediate action to improve police relations with minority groups. Fortunately, these business leaders were sufficiently concerned that they organized a nonprofit group called "Community Effort, Inc.", and obtained a charter enabling them to raise money for the operational funds of the program. Initially, the group raised $50,000 and followed that with a campaign to raise another $50,000. This money was used for the consulting psychologists' fees, for secretarial and clerical help, miscellaneous supplies, bussing of community participants and, for the first few laboratories, salaries of the participating police. Later in the program, the city assumed the responsibility for paying the officers for time spent in the group sessions. The total operating cost for one six-week session, accommodating 200 officers and an equal number of citizens, was approximately $20,000, of which sum, half went to police salaries.

Availability of private financial support meant that there was no federal intervention or control of the program. It also meant that it was an entirely local effort to combat a local problem. The absence of outside influence on both the direction and financing of the program made it more palatable to all concerned in deciding to give the program a trial. On October 9, 1967, the Houston Cooperative Crime Prevention Project officially began.

The Program Format — Human Relations Training

The model employed to serve as a structural and procedural guideline for conducting the police-community program was that provided by the Houston VA Hospital Human Relations Training Laboratory (Hanson, Rothaus, Johnson, & Lyle, 1966). This laboratory also supplied the police-community program with a majority of the group leaders experienced in human relations training. The Houston VA Human Relations Training Laboratory was founded in 1961, as an experiment in applying the concepts and techniques of the "T" group and sensitivity training approach to the problems of psychiatric patients. Departing from the traditional psychiatric treatment emphasis on the medical model, the training laboratory stresses a learning approach in the acquisition of new techniques to solve problems in living. This laboratory philosophy, emphasizing a problem centered experimental attitude toward the resolution of conflict, served as a conceptual guideline for the Houston police-community program. Techniques borrowed from psychodrama and sensitivity training, such as role reversal, "doubling", role mirroring, and "concentric circles", were employed as primary vehicles in the exchange of feelings between police and community.

The major goal of the police-community program (Sikes, 1967) was to:

> effect optimum interpersonal relationships among the various segments of the Houston community and those dedicated to the protection of the rights of these individuals — the police officers. More specifically, the program is designed to ease existing tension between law enforcement and minority groups — particularly the Negro and the Mexican-American. (p. 1)

In order to realize the general goal stated above, a more specific statement of the problem had to be considered so that its implementation, in terms of program design, could be carried out. The specific goals of the program were: first, to have the police and community groups examine the damaging stereotypes that they have of each other; second, to consider the extent to which these stereotypes affect their attitudes, perceptions, and behaviors, and ways they themselves reinforce these stereotypes in the eyes of the other group; and third, to develop a cooperative problem-solving attitude directed toward resolving differences and reducing conflict to a level where both groups could work together constructively. The planning group decided that the design needed to include some sort of face-to-face confrontation between community and police, in which both groups could express their feelings without fear of consequences.

Part of the staff, with the help of the Houston Council on Human Relations, concentrated on enlisting volunteers from the community to commit themselves to attend the six sessions within a series. Attempts were made to make this group as representative of the community as possible. The remaining staff, the group leaders, and representatives of the Police Academy[3] devoted their efforts to the program itself. Since it was impossible, because of personnel shortage, to have the police attend during their regular work hours, they were scheduled to come during their off duty hours, but in uniform.

---

[3]Particular credit is due Inspector C. D. Taylor, then Commanding Officer, Bureau of Personnel and Prevention, Houston Police Department, for his unceasing support of the Houston police-community program.

Program Design

The Houston police-community program contained nine phases to be completed in 6 three-hour blocks of time. Two hundred officers attended 1 three-hour session each week (40 policemen each day, five days per week) until the 18 hours were completed. At the completion of each 18-hour program, a new group of 200 policemen was enrolled until the entire force of approximately 1400 officers had completed the series. For each 18-hour series, an equal number of community members was sought with an attempt to make this group as representative of the community as possible. During the initial session, the police and community members were divided into three groups: three police and three community. Each of the six groups was assigned a group leader. Group leaders consisted primarily of psychologists, drawn from the staff of the Houston VA Hospital and the Departments of Psychology at TSU and the University of Houston, psychology trainees, and others who were experienced in group dynamics or techniques designed to facilitate change. Trainees in the VA Psychology Training Program with experience in group therapy and human relations training were employed as assistant group leaders.

Although the major framework of the design was set, group leaders implemented it in ways they felt would be most productive considering their own style and the nature of the population with which they were dealing. In addition to the group sessions, group leaders met every Friday afternoon to exchange ideas, suggest modifications, and share experiences.

The following paragraphs contain a phase-by-phase breakdown of the program and the approximate number of hours spent on each phase.

Phase I. Orientation

One hour was spent in orienting both groups to the program, its background design and goals. Community members were asked to make a commitment for the six weeks so that there would be some continuity within their group. Community members were also encouraged to ask questions to clear up any misconceptions about the program they might have gained from newspaper accounts. The officers were given a brief orientation lecture by a senior staff officer who emphasized the importance of the program for the welfare of the community and their need to participate wholeheartedly.

Phase II. Intragroup Development of Own Image and Image of Other

In the initial design, community members and police met separately during this phase to develop their own images and images of the other group.

This strategy was taken from a union-management conflict resolution described by Blake, Mouton, and Sloma (1965). Group members were first asked to make individual lists of the ways in which they saw themselves as a group. They were then asked to try to develop a group list, through consensus, about their own image. At the completion of this task, each group was then asked to develop a list of images of the other group. For the community members, this task was not very difficult. For the police group, however, it was an extremely complex task since they had to identify the segment of the community for which they were developing images.

The resulting self- and other images developed by the police and community groups are far too numerous to be listed. However, a summary of some of the more salient images will serve to present the flavor of this aspect of the group sessions.

Police self-image. As officers we are ethical, honest, physically clean and neat in appearance, and dedicated to our job, and we have a strong sense of duty. Some officers are prejudiced, but they are in the minority, and other officers are aware of their prejudice and so lean over backwards to be fair. We are a close knit, suspicious group, distrustful of outsiders. We put on a professional front: hard, calloused, and indifferent, but underneath, we have feelings. We treat others as nicely as they will let us. We are clannish, ostracized by the community, used as scapegoats, and under scrutiny even when off duty trying to enjoy ourselves. We are the blue minority.

Police image of community. Basically the public is cooperative and law-abiding, but uninformed about the duties, procedures, and responsibilities of the police officer. The rich, upper-class person is supportive of the police, but feels immune to the law and uses his money and influence to avoid police action against himself and his children. The middle-class person is supportive of the police and more civic minded than the upper or lower classes. The major share of police contact with the middle class is through traffic violations. The lower-class person has the most frequent contact with the police and usually is uncooperative as a witness or in reporting crime. He has a different sense of values; he lives only for today and doesn't plan for tomorrow. As police officers, we see the Houston Negro in two groups: (1) Negro — industrious, productive, moral, law-abiding, and not prone to violence; (2) "nigger" — lazy, immoral, dishonest, unreliable, and prone to violence.

Community self-image. We lack knowledge about proper police procedures and do not know our rights, obligations, and duties in regard to the law. There is a lack of communication among social, geographical, racial, and economic segments of the community. We don't involve ourselves in civic affairs as we should, and we have guilty consciences about the little crimes (traffic violations) we get away with, but are resentful when caught. We relate to the police as authority figures, and we feel uncomfortable around them. The black community feels itself to be second class in relation to the police. The majority of the community are law-abiding, are hard working, pay taxes, and are honest and reliable.

Community image of police. Some police abuse their authority by acting as judge, jury, and prosecutor, and assuming a person to be guilty until proven innocent. Too often the police are psychologically and physically abusive; they indulge in name-calling, handle people roughly, and discriminate against blacks in applying the law. The police are cold and mechanical in the performance of their duties. They see the world only through their squad car windshields and are walled off from the community. We expect them to be perfect, to make no mistakes, and to set the standards for behavior. Our initial reaction when we see an officer is "blue."

Phases III and IV. Exchange and Clarification of Images

Police and community members met in face-to-face confrontation groups to exchange and clarify the images each had developed of the other. These images were reproduced and a list was distributed to all members. The major task during these phases was to have the members of each group clarify what they meant by the images they had developed. The purpose was not to assess the accuracy of the image, but merely to clarify it. It was extremely difficult to keep both groups focused on the task. Each group would frequently become defensive and deny the reality of the other's perceptions. During these two phases, many heated exchanges occurred. Group leaders were focusing on process and using techniques to facilitate this exchange and clarification. Role playing, psychodrama, group observations, lecturettes, and other devices borrowed from the fields of human relations training and group therapy were employed by the group leaders. Three hours were devoted to these phases.

Phases V and VI. Intragroup Diagnosis of Present Relationship and Exchange of These Diagnoses Across Groups

During the intragroup diagnosis, the community and police met separately for one hour. Their task was to look at their own behaviors in terms of how they were stereotyped by the other group, and to explore how these behaviors facilitated the image the other group held of them. Each group made a list of these behaviors; this list was reproduced and distributed to all members. Police and community members met again for the remaining two hours of the session to share these diagnoses. In some cases, group leaders did not divide the police and community groups, but had them observe each other as they attempted to diagnose their own behaviors. Both groups had a tendency to return to the previous confrontation phase and had to be brought back to the task. This was particularly true of community members who were present for the first time or who had missed the first few sessions.

Phase VII. Identification of Key Issues and Sources of Friction

During this phase, attempts were made to get the community and police to work cooperatively in a problem-solving manner. To facilitate this, some group leaders divided the entire group into two or three smaller groups, each consisting of both community members and police. This procedure tended to reduce their identity as separate groups. The problem each group had was to look back over the previous sessions and try to come up with a list of key issues that tended to keep the community and police divided. On the basis of the images, the intragroup diagnoses, and the community-police interaction during the program, several areas or barriers to communication were usually identified.

Phase VIII. Planning Steps to Alleviate Sources of Friction and Making Recommendations

Approximately three to four hours were spent on this phase. Both police and community members worked cooperatively, devising ways in which the key decisive issues could be alleviated. Again, there were occasional regressions to the confrontation phase among the community members.

Phase IX. Evaluation

The last phase was devoted to some discussion of the value of the whole program. In addition, instruments were devised to elicit participants' reactions to the program as a whole, and to comment on what value the program had for them in their work as police officers, or in their roles as citizens. For some of the sessions, evaluations were made on a pre- and post-treatment basis in order to study attitudinal change. These findings will be discussed in the section on evaluation.

Design Problems and Modifications

Community Attendance

In order to implement the design as presented, it was important to have continuity of attendance from both groups. Since the police were required to attend, this problem did not arise with them. The community members, however, were inconsistent in their attendance. Images that would be developed by a group during one week frequently had to be handled and explained by another group the following week. That is, community dropouts from each session would be replaced by new members in the following session. During the entire six weeks there was a core of community members whose attendance was consistent. A large number, however, were either inconsistent or were entering the program at any phase during a series. As a consequence, it was difficult to predict who would comprise the community representation from week to week.

In addition, it was difficult to get a cross section of the community. During the first three series there was a predominance of lower socio-economic groups. Most of these were from the Negro community. Special efforts were made to get representative samples from other groups, particularly Mexican-American. This problem was somewhat alleviated by obtaining intact groups from organizations in the community who would commit themselves for the six weeks.

Clarity of Goals

In the original Blake and Mouton (1965) design, both management and union leaders had the same goals, e.g., increased production. It was extremely difficult, in the present program, to determine to what extent the goals of the community and the police were consistent. For example, the motivation of some community members for attending was primarily to air their grievances against the police, but not necessarily to solve mutual problems. Some members from both police and community were probably more interested in perpetuating the conflict than in alleviating it, i.e., carrying the confrontation phase into the later phases. As a whole, however, it was fairly clear that both police and community did not want to perpetuate the conflict.

Another implicit goal that seemed to be clouding the issue was the attempt of each group to change the other. When this was evident, both groups responded more defensively. Both groups felt freer to acknowledge their own problems and need for change when they were not pressured by the other group to do so.

Many attempts were made through the newspapers and the television to get community members to attend these sessions. The presentation of the purpose of these meetings, however, was not always consistent with the goals as stated above. The purpose was often presented as an opportunity for community members to air their grievances against the police. With this in mind, many community members attended primarily to criticize the police department. As a consequence, many policemen may have felt that they were being scapegoated for the benefit of the community. The orientation meetings, however, restated the goals of the program so that this discrepancy in presentation was somewhat alleviated.

Confrontation Without Problem Solving

After the first few series, many of the group leaders modified the initial design and concentrated more on the face-to-face confrontations of the two groups. Most of the group leaders made some attempt during the last few sessions to have community and police groups work cooperatively on solving the problems dividing them. Other leaders attempted to resolve issues as they arose throughout the series. A few group leaders, however, allowed the community and the police to continue to confront each other for all six sessions. As a consequence, these community members and police officers did not have the experience of working *together* to resolve their differences. Thus many of the group members from both sides finished the series without any closure. Because new community members entered the groups each week, continuous confrontation without resolution was an ever present problem that had to be dealt with by the leaders.

Pretraining Police Groups

The extent to which both community and police were defensive soon became obvious to the group leaders. In addition, it was apparent that although many policemen have differed with their fellow officers on certain issues, they did not feel free to air these feelings. There appeared to be pressure within the police group to present a solid front. As a consequence, many disagreements *within* the police group did not get expressed. This pressure to conform was not as great among the community members who were not related to each other in any work situation and, therefore, had less to lose by disagreeing with other community members. Some pretraining for the police in terms of their own attitudes and feelings toward each other and some focus on process issues rather than content might have enabled the police to be more productive in these confrontation meetings. That is, they might have been less defensive about their own problem areas and felt freer to disagree with each other in front of the community.

Randomizing Groups

Although there were attempts by the police officials to randomize the selection of police officers in terms of openness to the program, length of time in service, and rank, there were several police groups that seemed to be very negatively biased toward the program. These groups were most difficult to work with because there were little or no resources in the group to counter the hostile and negative attitudes. In addition, these and other groups (those meeting mostly during the working day hours) were further disappointed and frustrated by the fact that it was extremely difficult to recruit community members for these sessions. Many of the officers felt that there was no point in meeting if there were not going to be any community members present.

Evaluation of Program Effectiveness

Problems of Evaluation

Many of the problems attendant on the organization and operation of a community action program, such as the Houston police-community project, also confound program evaluation. Administration of attitude scales or other psychological instruments requires cooperation and motivation on the part of the respondents. It is hardly necessary to point out that, in the present project, a ready supply of the traditional, bright, and eager psychology research subjects was not available (i.e., the proverbial college sophomores, who can be persuaded to respond to any psychological device or evaluation instrument placed before them). Instead, we were confronted with two antagonistic groups, suspicious of each other, of their surroundings, of the program administrators and leaders, and paranoid about the purpose and goals of the program itself.

Psychologists usually pursue their scientific careers aided by the luxury of having as a subject, the college sophomore, who is required by departmental rule to serve in research as a condition for enrolling in psychology. This research subject responds eagerly when the MMPI, a self-concept test, Rorschach cards, or a battery of social values inventories are thrust under his nose. Ideally, this type of pre- and post-testing should have been included in the project, together with periodic post-treatment follow-up evaluation. In addition, matched police and community groups who did not go through the program, but who were similarly evaluated as control groups, should have been studied.

Unfortunately, this scientific ideal had to give way to what was possible and practical. There would have been little gained if, in the process of imposing on our subjects an intrusive evaluation procedure, the project itself were destroyed.

The atmosphere surrounding the program can be further delineated by noting that the first groups met in the Police Academy. It was taken for granted by the police that the room was wired and that whatever transpired would be recorded. This wasn't even a topic for discussion by the police, but was merely accepted as a component of the air they breathed. Community members attending many of the group meetings refused even to wear name tags during the group sessions, fearing that they would be identified by the police and later, if they said anything derogatory, be recriminated against. Some community participants had previous convictions or were currently under indictment for alleged crimes. Naturally, they wanted to remain anonymous.

At the outset, the police tended to view the program as designed only to provide disgruntled and complaining citizens a chance to criticize and berate them. Officers were particularly suspicious of those group leaders regularly employed by the federal government, as if they represented agents of a foreign power. Community members questioned the motives of those responsible for originating the program, fearing that the hidden purpose of the program was to reduce them to docile lackeys of "the Establishment." As the program progressed, it attracted national attention and the interest of the news media. The American Broadcasting Company prepared a one-hour TV "special" based on the program and, without the knowledge or permission of the staff, chose to title the presentation, "Prejudice and the Police — a program designed to detect racial prejudice among members of the Houston Police Department." Needless to say, such a distortion did nothing to improve police acceptance of the program.

Other factors limiting the kind of tests or questionnaires that could be employed included the fleeting cooperation and concentration span for both police and community participants. In addition, some community members were either illiterate or non-English and, judging from their poor handwriting, grammar, and spelling, some of the police had rather limited verbal skills.

Post-Treatment Evaluation

Faced with this discouraging array of limitations as to possible avenues of evaluation, it soon became evident that no psychological instrument existed that fulfilled the requisites for this program: brief, subtle, simple and easy to administer, nonthreatening, and yielding results meaningful to the present investigation. Moreover, it was clear that if the project was inaugurated by thrusting an MMPI under the nose of the police or the community, the program might collapse before it had begun.

Accordingly, the evaluation began on a modest note. A brief anonymous questionnaire was devised, one for police and one for community, that was administered at the close of the final or sixth session. This questionnaire asked for an overall rating of the program on a poor to excellent scale, and asked, as well, for an indication of whether attitudes toward the police or community had changed as a result of the program. The findings of an earlier report by Sikes and Cleveland (1968, p. 767) are listed in Table II, where the response to these questions by about 800 of the city's 1400 man police force and 600 participating citizens is presented. As can be seen, community acceptance is strongly positive, with police reaction moderately good.

Table II

Police-Community Response to a Human Relations Training Laboratory

Rating	% Police	% Community
Excellent	4	18
Very good	23	33
Good	58	42
Poor	15	7
Feelings more positive	37	65
Feelings more negative	2	4
Feelings unchanged	61	31

Note: This table and the analysis of police and community reaction to the program is reprinted from *The American Psychologist* (Sikes & Cleveland, 1968), by permission of The American Psychological Association.

Other items on the questionnaire inquired as to the course impact on understanding of police and community problems and relationships. Analysis of the spontaneous comments noted by police and community participants on their evaluation sheets in response to these questions provides the following summary of areas of attitude change effected by the program.

Police

1. The police are gratified that the community has gained some appreciation of the policeman's role, of what he can do and cannot do. The police seemed surprised as to how misinformed the public is regarding police procedures, the limits of their authority, and the nature of their duties. This is best expressed by a policeman who noted on his evaluation sheet: "I wasn't aware that the community was so misinformed as to my duties. They expect the police department to answer every problem, for example, as to marking streets or building bridges."

2. It was recognized that the police may provoke situations and aggravate feelings by verbal abuse, the use of "trigger" words ("boy," "nigger," "Spic," etc.). Some policemen realized that they can unintentionally hurt others by this name-calling. For example, an officer commented, "As a policeman, I have learned how defensive we really are — how much I rationalize. I have learned that we can hurt people without really knowing it."

3. The police became aware of, and in some instances were shocked by, the intensity of the hatred for the police among some community members. Among some officers, this confrontation served as an eye-opener regarding the intensity of antipolice feelings within the Negro community. One officer put it this way in his evaluation notes: "I didn't realize there was as strong a resentment against the Police Department as some people of the Negro community expressed." Another said, "I never realized so many people had such deep resentment toward the police. It made me stop and think."

4. There is a massive defensiveness among the police as to any wrongdoing on their part, and as to any need for change in their attitudes or behavior. There is also a pretty general feeling that to admit to misbehavior is to admit to weakness and failure. This majority position is offset, to some extent, by an expressed recognition among a minority of the police of their defensiveness and need to deny or excuse misbehavior on the part of officers. This defensiveness is represented in the following statement made by one officer: "I feel the entire course should have been eliminated. There was nothing brought out that was not known. Nothing was said to change my opinions. All the community wants is the police to give in to them." But a more open attitude is represented in opinions expressed by a minority of the officers, in statements such as: "The course has caused me to see myself as the community sees me. It has brought to light things which I did not think the public was even aware of."

5. The program resulted in some awareness of the need to control personal feelings and emotions and to respond in a courteous and self-controlled manner. One officer commented: "It made me understand that although I may have preconceived ideas or biased opinions of people, that I must strive as a policeman to keep these out of my personal dealings with others. I should go further to understand what might motivate this person to feel the way they do (sic)."

Community

1. There is a greater awareness of policeman's role, his problems, and scope of his responsibilities as well as a better understanding of police procedures as to why officers ask certain questions, issue certain orders, and often appear brusque, indifferent, and even rude and insensitive. One community member put it this way: "This course will bring a better

understanding between the policeman and myself to the community which I reside in and through this understanding there will be more cooperation in feeling that he, the policeman, will get respect and, as citizens, we will realize more that he is doing his job."

2. Citizens recognized their responsibilities to promote law and order, to "become involved," and to work *with* and not against or apart from the police. For example, one citizen commented: "This course has enabled me to understand the duties and responsibilities of the police and how we, the community, can cooperate with them in doing a better job." Another said, "I was never fully aware of the many problems facing the police in their duties and how the community tends to hinder the police, instead of helping. As a community, we fail to get involved when we should."

3. There is greater respect for the police as individual human beings rather than as members of one undifferentiated group, the "blue minority." Citizens came to recognize their tendency to view the police as authoritarian robots, rather than real people who sometimes make honest mistakes, get angry, and behave unwisely. Police were seen as unfeeling and lacking in sympathy. Some citizens commented upon completion of the course: "Before this course I regarded the policeman as a symbol of authority, not as a real human being." "The community sometimes reacts blindly against policemen as a whole. I could see that a great many police want to do a good job in a professional manner." "The police officer has become, for me, more a human being and less of a sadistic robot."

4. There is a recognition by community members of their own bias and prejudice toward the police. This point was illustrated well in one citizen's evaluation of his response to the program: "I find that I possess a good deal of hostility, and prejudged and preconceived notions and ideas toward the police, which were incorporated into my personality before I attended these meetings."

5. Citizens expressed the hope that some of the police will change their behavior and attitudes toward minority group members. There is a note of optimism that there will be change for the better, which replaces the feeling of despair that nothing will change.

6. Some community members developed at least an intellectual understanding of how their attitudes and feelings can influence and shape their perception of reality, their view of the police and police behavior.

7. Citizens felt a sense of freedom and release in the opportunity to criticize, talk back to, yell at, and challenge the statement of a policeman without retaliation or fear of retribution.

8. There developed an understanding of some of the pressures the police feel subjected to — shortage of personnel, personal risk and danger, inferior and obsolete equipment, internal friction, and archaic rules within the police department. One community member stated, "This course has helped in

understanding the problems of the police, how they jeopardize their lives, and the apathy they must deal with."

9. It was recognized by many community members that they tended to demand of the police ideal and perfect behavior. One community member expressed the sentiment of many in commenting on his evaluation sheet, "I now recognize that policemen are human beings who may make mistakes instead of machines that should never make a mistake."

10. Fear of police as threatening authority figures was reduced. This was expressed by one community member who scrawled on his evaluation sheet, "It (the course) has taken away the fear."

There is a footnote to be added to this report on community response to the program. One of the six-week sessions was devoted almost exclusively to Latin American community participants and the meetings were held in the predominantly Latin American neighborhoods. Among the Latin Americans there was an overwhelming acceptance of the program, with nearly every participant rating it as "Excellent", no one rating the program less than "very good" and unanimous agreement that the program had resulted in more positive feelings toward the police. The extent to which the police are viewed with awe and reverence by the Latin-Americans in a kind of humble genuflection to authority, is further illustrated in one summary provided by a participant, writing in Spanish, regarding his perception of the policeman: "The police is the guardian of our society, like the priest is of his church. He is the guide of our souls. The uniform does not indicate fear, but respect. He is the defender or the representative of law and justice."

Pre- and Post-Treatment Evaluation

After the project had been underway for several months, the program staff felt more secure in imposing on the police pre- and post-evaluation of their attitudes. A 31-item questionnaire (later expanded to 38 items) was then developed, called the "Community Attitude Survey" (CAS), designed to evaluate attitudes toward the poor, minority groups, and the community at large. All scale items are presented in Likert format, with provision for checking each response on a six-point continuum from strongly agree to strongly disagree. Most of the items were constructed from comments made by the police on their evaluation sheets. Some items were adapted from the Cohen-Struening Opinions About Mental Illness scale (Cohen & Struening, 1962) and a couple of items were adapted from the F scale.

The 31 CAS items were evaluated according to several criteria. This was done on two samples of police participants. The first sample of 148 Ss responded to the questionnaire following their completion of the program (Group 1). A second sample of 120 police was surveyed upon their entry into the program (Group 2), and again, six weeks later, on completion of the course. The responses to each item of these two groups were submitted to a principal axis factor analysis with varimax rotation. Originally, 10 rotated factors were extracted for each group, but this solution was not very satisfactory because of the number of ill-defined factors and the lack of correspondence in the two groups. Rotation of only the first four factors proved a more stable, interpretable solution; it accounted for 37% of the variance in Group 1, and 38% in Group 2.

In computing factor scores based on this analysis, an item was assigned to a factor if it had an average loading for the two samples of roughly .35 or higher. Each item thus selected had a weight of one in the composite factor score. The four factors thus obtained were:

Factor I, *Minority Group Prejudice*, loaded on 16 items and accounted for the greater percentage of variance (14 and 16% in the two groups). The items were characterized by depreciatory attitudes toward minority or poverty groups, in which lower standards and unfavorable characteristics were attributed to them. Some items with the highest loadings were: "People in poverty areas don't really care how they live." "Poor people are lazy and don't really want to work." "If people in poverty areas were provided nice homes they would soon turn them into slums." "When minority groups complain, they just want to gripe and make trouble." This last item is related to another aspect of the factor, the denial of justifiable complaints on the part of minority group members. A corollary set of items with lower loadings involves refusal to concede the possibility of reason, understanding, and humane treatment in relation to minority or "underclass" groups, e.g., "It doesn't do any good to talk things over with people from minority groups because all they understand is force."

Factor II, *Disrespect for the Law*, represents the feeling that the community lacks respect for the law and appreciation of its representatives, the police. There were five items in this factor such as: "People in the community don't understand what the police have to put up with." "Most of all this country needs more respect for law and order."

Factor III, *Class Discrimination*, comprises five items which compare lower class members directly and unfavorably with higher status groups. There is an implication that people should be judged and treated differentially on the basis of their social status. Examples of items are: "You have to judge the behavior of people living in poverty areas by different standards than those living in better parts of the city." "Juvenile delinquency is found mostly in lower-class, minority groups." "It is all right for a respectable citizen to possess a gun, but unwise to let people in poverty areas have them."

Factor IV, *Police-Community Images*, loads on five items and is probably the weakest in terms of interpretability. Three of the items relate to the perception of community feelings about the police; e.g., "Most people respect and appreciate the police." The other two refer to discriminatory attitudes toward different classes in the community; e.g., "Generally speaking there are two kinds of people: respectable citizens and law-breakers."

A large number of items, (20 in all) had substantial loadings on the first unrotated factor of the principal axis solution. This may be taken as a general factor representing a prejudiced, unfavorable attitude toward minority groups and the poor (*General Prejudice*). Items with average loadings of about .35 or higher were scored on this general factor. Most of these items loaded on Factors I and II of the rotated analysis. As an additional criterion for a general attitude common to the CAS, each item was correlated with a total score based on 31 items definitely capable of being scored as to prejudice. For Police Group 1, 27 items had correlations of .21 or better, significant at the .01 level. Of these, 20 had an *r* of .40 or higher. In a student group of 68 *S*s, this same criterion yielded 24 items significant at the .01 level, which required an *r* of .31. Again, 20 items had an *r* of .40 or better. With few exceptions, correlations in the two groups were of similar magnitude. Loadings on the students' first principal axis factor were also consistent with the police results. However, the rotated factor structure for the students showed little correspondence to the police samples beyond the first factor. When the item means of the police and students were compared by F-test, 24 items discriminated the two groups at the .01 level. Of the seven which failed to do so, five had a low, nonsignificant relationship to the total prejudice score and to the general factor.

In brief, the CAS demonstrated fair stability of factor composition for police groups when a limited number of orthogonal factors were extracted. The criterion of internal consistency showed that most items correlated significantly with an overall score and loaded substantially on a general (first principal axis) factor. These same items also correlated with total score for college students, and showed substantial, significant differences between student and police means.

Pre- and post-testing of the police presented some problems since it was desirable to identify individual responses on a before and after basis. However, the Police Department did not want either the officers' real names or a code list used for identification. An attempt was made to identify the individual pre- and post-questionnaires by having the police put their age and years on force on both questionnaires. However, some officers deliberately altered their stated age and years on force, changed their handwriting style, or left these items blank in an effort to defeat our investigation. For this particular class of officers, 120 valid pre-test questionnaires were obtained and 90 post-tests, or 75% of the original sample. Some officers did not attend the final group session when the post-testing was accomplished and some apparently failed to hand in the questionnaire. Of the 90 valid post-tests obtained, it was possible to match 84 with a corresponding pre-test.

Comparison of pre- vs. post-test means for the four factors on the CAS plus the general prejudice score is made in Table III. It will be noted that all post-test means are lower, or in the direction of less prejudice. Differences for Factors I and II, *Minority Group Prejudice* and *Disrespect for the Law*, are significant at the .05 level of confidence. For the *General Prejudice* score and Factor IV, *Police-Community Images*, the pre- vs. post-test mean score difference attains significance at the .01 level. Only Factor III, *Class Discrimination*, fails to change significantly.

Table III

Police Pre- and Post-CAS Factor Scores

	Factor I	Factor II	Factor III	Factor IV	General Prejudice
Pre-test mean	49.33	12.02	4.55	16.93	74.61
Post-test mean	46.71	10.92	4.29	15.82	71.35
t (related means)	2.30	2.61	.54	2.65	2.69
P(df=82)	.05	.05	NS	.01	.01

Although these attitudinal changes on the part of the police attain a level of statistical significance, it is uncertain how much practical meaning this may have. With groups of this size only a small consistent shift in scores is needed to achieve statistical significance. Whether these modest changes are also translated into meaningful alterations in the officers' perception of poverty and minority groups is open to question. At the very least, a measurable, although minimal, shift in attitude seemed to have been achieved, following 18 hours of confrontation with the community.

As has been mentioned, a group of 148 officers were administered the CAS on a postlaboratory basis only and their scores compared with those of 68 college students. The students and police differed significantly (.01 level) on 24 of the 31 items, with the police scoring in the direction of more expressed prejudice. Of course, the student and police groups differ with respect to age, sex, education, and other important demographic variables. This comparison is reported only to illustrate that groups with differing composition do respond in a contrasting manner on the CAS.

For this same group of 148 officers, and contrary to our expectations, there was no relationship between the *General Prejudice* score and either chronological age or years on force. Age correlated .04 with prejudice score, and years on force, .03.

Subsequent Pre-Post Evaluation

Comparison of police vs. community attitudes. At this point in the program, the investigators were congratulating themselves on the modest degree of success achieved in altering attitudes following exposure to an 18-hour dialogue. Community acceptance of the program had already been demonstrated to be enthusiastic and police response was at least grudgingly accepting.

However, evaluation of the next police-community session altered the rosy picture conjectured by the investigators. The CAS was again administered on a pre- and post-program basis, this time to both the officers and citizens in attendance. The original 31-item CAS was enlarged to 38 items for this administration, with the deletion of one item from the old form and the addition of eight new items.

The officers drew numbers from a hat and were asked to record this number on both their pre- and post-CAS questionnaires. Valid questionnaires were obtained for 100 officers on the pre-testing. However, only 57 post-tests could be matched, as many officers left their post-tests unidentified or put the same number on more than one test. One officer identified his post-test with the notation, "Full fledged member KKK," and another by sketching a man hanging from a scaffold.

For the community, 160 valid pre-tests were obtained. Unfortunately, community participation in this laboratory session was not consistent and it was not possible to obtain a representative sample of post-tests from the same citizens on whom pre-tests were available. Accordingly, pre- and post-evaluation of community response to the CAS could not be made.

Comparison of the responses of 100 officers and 160 citizens on whom pre-test CAS scores were available reveals that police and community differ beyond the .01 level on 36 of the 38 items, with the police in each case scoring at the high prejudice end of the scale. While it is not surprising that the police and predominantly black community differ in their attitudes on social issues, the scope and intensity of their dissidence underline the conceptual and philosophical chasm separating these groups.

For example, the police and community differ most sharply on the following items, with the mean police response in each case agreeing with the statement and the community flatly disagreeing:

"Anyone willing to work can get a suitable job today."

"The main cause of riots and civil disorders is disrespect for the law."

"A few professional agitators are causing all our social unrest. If it weren't for them there would be no trouble."

"If people in poverty areas were provided nice homes, they would soon turn them into slums."

"Very few real problems exist between the police and community in Houston."

Pre- and post-evaluation of police attitudes. It was possible to match only 57 post-test police questionnaires with 100 obtained pre-tests. As has been mentioned, officers frequently failed to place an identification number on their post-tests or put the same number on more than one test, invalidating the pre-/post-comparison.

Factor analysis of the revised 38-item CAS for this group of officers revealed that a major source of the variance rested with the *General Prejudice* score. This group differed in this respect from other police groups and from their own pre-test response on the CAS, with nearly all items loading on the unrotated factor (*General Prejudice*). For example, this factor accounted for 35% of the total variance on the post-testing compared to only 24% on the pre-testing for this group of officers. This is also in contrast with the first police group on whom pre- and post-CAS tests were obtained, where the *General Prejudice* score accounted for only 18% of the total variance on pre-testing and 22% on post-testing.

Because of this polarization of attitudes among these officers, further analysis of the CAS scores for the four special factors was not attempted. It was found that for the 57 officers on whom pre- and post-tests were available there was a significant (.01 level) *increase* in *General Prejudice* score from pre- to post-testing.

In other words, only about half the officers in this group were willing to identify their postlaboratory attitudes, even when using a code number, known only to them. Of those cooperating, an increase, rather than a decrease, in expressed prejudice was obtained following 18 hours of intercourse with the community, which was intended to reduce bias. Examination of the post-test questionnaires revealed that many officers simply chose the most extreme response for every test item. Even several "lie" items on the scale were rejected by the officers. For example, the item, "People living in poverty areas deserve as much respect and kind treatment as anyone else", a sentiment previous police groups had uniformly agreed to, was marked "strongly disagree" by many officers in this group.

How can these unforeseen and contradictory results be explained? Why did attitudes become crystallized at the extreme prejudice end of the scale following this particular community relations program? Most likely, the explanation lies in events occurring outside the framework of the program and the introduction of social forces much more powerful than those generated by the police-community exchange itself. One such force was the systematic attendance at these group sessions of white members of an extreme right wing political group who participated as community representatives. Their attendance culminated in a detailed article on the program appearing in a local newspaper with strong right-wing political bias. This article described the "brain washing" techniques, self-criticism, and confessional approaches used by the "Communist Revolution" and left the reader with the impression that the police-community program was similar in goals and procedure. The program was portrayed as part of a nationwide conspiracy to subvert law enforcement agencies. The article enjoyed wide circulation within the police department. During the coffee break, these same community participants also distributed to the officers in their group a pamphlet entitled, *Hate Therapy*, which described sensitivity training as a systematic effort on the part of the "far left" to impose world rule on mankind.

A second and probably even more telling event was the clash between Chicago police and demonstrators associated with the National Democratic Convention. This event served to polarize attitudes in a dramatic fashion and probably was largely responsible for inspiring the negative response of the police in recording their attitudes on the post-testing which occurred only one week after the Chicago disturbance. It was reported (*Houston Chronicle*, 1968) that 300 Houston officers sent a collective telegram to the Chicago police department supporting and praising the police action there. The post-test administration of the CAS, coming so soon after the Chicago incident while feelings were still running high, probably served as a convenient medium for the police in expressing their frustrations on the issue of law and order. This would account for their polarization of attitudes on the CAS, a phenomenon not noted in earlier groups.

Later Program Evaluation

Consistent community attendance on a voluntary basis for 18 hours over a six-week period proved to be an intolerable burden on community participants. Recognizing this, later laboratory sessions were shortened to four weeks in the hopes of securing more consistent community participation. In addition, groups were reduced in size to 7 officers and 7-10 community members, with community membership closed after the first session, in the hopes of building more cohesive groups that would generate their own group loyalty and member identification, thus assuring more regular community attendance.

Evaluation of one of these shortened laboratories indicates increased community participation and much less resistance displayed by participating officers. The CAS was administered to 62 officers and 105 community members on a posttreatment only basis. Pre- and post-evaluation was not attempted in view of previous difficulties encountered in identification of the questionnaires.

This group of officers differs significantly from the previous group of 57 officers on six of the CAS items, with the officers who participated in the more recent abbreviated laboratory making consistently lower prejudice scores than those officers who went through the six-week program. This finding suggests greater program impact for the abbreviated session, although no definitive conclusion can be reached since pre- and post-studies were not available.

Earlier community and police participants had differed on 36 of the 38 CAS items, with the police having higher prejudice scores. Comparison of the 105 community members and 62 officers participating in the shortened seminar reveals significant differences on only 26 of the 38 items on the CAS. In fact, the officers and citizens in this group actually differ sharply on only nine of the items, i.e., where the officers agree and citizens flatly disagree with an item. These findings suggest that this group of officers and citizens may have drawn closer together in their social views following their four-week interchange.

Evaluation of the last police-community session, marking the conclusion of the program, was accomplished by reverting to the brief questionnaire used in the initial sessions. While there was some shift in police and community attitudes about the program as compared to the early sessions, the overall response was largely unchanged (see Table II). For example, 79% of this final police class rate the program somewhere between good and excellent; 21% rate it poor. Also, 35% say their community attitudes are more positive following the program; 61% say their feelings are unchanged. For the community, 90% rate the program good to excellent and 65% say their attitudes toward the police are more positive, with 30% unchanged.

Paper and pencil role playing. Finally, an attempt was made to evaluate attitude change among the police using a different procedure than the CAS questionnaire approach. In effect, the police were asked to do some paper and pencil role playing. Items were provided that invited the police to record their feelings in reaction to three hypothetical situations. The first item asked the officer to imagine himself, not as a policeman, but instead as a poor unemployed Negro. He was asked to write down as many different statements he could as to how he thought a policeman would appear to him under these conditions. A second item asked the officer to list as many arguments as he could supporting the following statement: "Some people believe that minority group members (Negroes, Latin-Americans, etc.) are naturally dull, lazy, and unwilling to help themselves." A third item asked for arguments supporting this proposition: "Other people feel that minority groups would be as successful and self-supporting as anyone else if they had the same educational, social, and job opportunities."

These items were included as a final sheet on the CAS questionnaire just described, and administered to the same police classes on a pre- and post-treatment basis. It was hoped that a simple count of the number of supporting statements elicited before and after the program might provide a measure of attitude change. Unfortunately, this type of evaluation was not very fruitful. Only about half the responding police recorded anything meaningful in response to these items. About 40% left the items blank and another 10% either misinterpreted the statements or failed to record anything relevant. This procedure was dropped from subsequent evaluations.

Among those policemen responding to these items in a meaningful way, there are one or two findings of interest. First of all, the officers are more proficient in finding arguments to support proposition two, the negative view of minority groups, than they are in supporting proposition three, which asks for positive statements about Negroes and Latin-Americans. However, on the post-testing, the number of arguments supporting the negative proposition declines, while the number of statements supporting the positive viewpoint remains unchanged. While the mean number of negative statements exceeds the positive on the pre-testing, the mean number of positive statements exceeds the negative on the post-testing, although not to a significant extent.

Empirical validity. Fortunately, evaluation of the effectiveness of this community action program in promoting better relationships between police and community members does not rest exclusively on the indirect evidence provided by response to questionnaires. It is possible to identify certain movements within the community suggestive of lessened tension between citizens and police. For one thing there has been no further rioting, and neither the assassination of Martin Luther King, Jr. nor of Robert F. Kennedy was followed by racial incidents. Another encouraging sign is that the Mayor's office reports a 70% reduction in citizen complaints about police behavior for the seven-month period following inception of the program (Justice, 1968). Finally, there are indications of subtle and quiet improvements in relationships: a white police officer organizes his own group of blacks and whites for continuing discussions in his home; officers stop their squad cars to talk with black people in their neighborhood, for no other reason than to meet them. Such incidents may be only straws in a climate of change and may, in fact, be due to forces entirely apart from the police-community program, but they do suggest change at the all-important behavioral level.

Reflections on a Community Action Program

A remark was made at one of the program staff meetings to the effect that, by the time this police-community project was finally terminated, the staff probably would have learned enough to be able to devise and conduct such a program properly. Certainly the program served as a learning experience, not only for the police and community participants, but for the staff as well. The following are some of the important structural, procedural, and administrative aspects of such a program, the proper and most effective handling of which was learned the hard way. These considerations are offered for perusal by personnel planning any such endeavor.

Administrative considerations. In order for any community action program to be successful, it must from the very start have full and open support from the responsible city officials. Grudging approval, innuendos about the program, and anything less than enthusiastic and wholehearted backing of the program by all administrative levels within the city administration will be detected by the participants and used by some as a basis for refusing to cooperate or become involved.

The professional staff recruited for such a program must resist pressures created by impending community crises to initiate a hastily assembled crash program. Because of tensions within the city, and the need created by this tension, the directors of the Houston program were catapulted into action before the kind of groundwork necessary for an effectively functioning program could be attempted. There was pressure from city officials to initiate something quickly and although the program directors protested that ample time was needed to think through the philosophy and goals of the program, as well as the methodology and myriad of operational details, the city fathers felt that an immediate beginning was mandatory. A dry run or trial laboratory to test out the effectiveness of alternate procedures would have been helpful. Another consequence of this precipitous organization was that neither the community nor the police officers were given an opportunity to involve themselves in the construction of the program. In retrospect, it is realized that representatives from both the police department and the community should have been consulted at the planning stage. Instead, the program was handed to them as a finished product. Perhaps if representatives of the police and community had participated in the planning of the program, both groups would have felt a greater involvement and a greater responsibility in seeing it through. This was particularly true for the police, who had to accept this assignment as they did any other order issued by their superiors.

The goals of a community action program should be clearly delineated and understood at the outset by those involved. These goals should be stated explicitly, so that later there is no misunderstanding as to what the project is attempting to accomplish. In the Houston project, the expectations for the accomplishments of the program were initially quite modest. The staff, as well as the supporters of the program, would have been willing to consider it a success if the participants, after an initial confrontation and exchange of images and attitudes, evidenced only slight shifts in their views of each other. However, the aspiration level for the program was raised as the project unfolded and attracted local, state, and national attention through television and news media coverage. There is a constant danger that the original modest goals for a community action program gradually may expand to an unrealistic degree, so that the project becomes a panacea for the social ills of a community. The Houston police-community program is now often pointed to as an example of Houston's progressiveness in community-police relations. Obscured is the lack of progressiveness that gave rise to the need for such a program.

Financial considerations. One would assume that if money were made available for an innovative police-community relations program, the major obstacle to initiating such a program would be cleared. For the present project, the availability of supporting funds only marked the onset of problems. It was necessary to resort to private philanthropy, since money from the federal government is regarded by many in Houston as if it came from a foreign, subversive power. For reasons of their own, the business leaders who contributed to the financial support of the program chose to remain anonymous, an action that later caused problems. Some police officers remained convinced that the financial backing for the program was either communist inspired, or a federal grant offered in an attempt to intervene in local affairs. On the other hand, many community members felt that the police department and the city were backing the program financially, that the purpose of the program was to reduce the community participants to the status of lackeys of the "Establishment", and that the group leaders were stooges of the police and the city administration. Explanations to the contrary often fell on deaf ears and individuals believed what they wanted to believe. Questions raised by the community and the police about the financial arrangements revolved about such issues as: "Who are the donors?" "Why are they doing this?" "What do *they* want to get out of this?" Failure to make explicit the financial structure of the program also created hardships for the group leaders, who felt defensive because they were also in the dark and could not answer questions posed by the officers and citizens regarding the origins of financial support for the program. Their own defensiveness on this point tended to increase distrust by the community and police group members. Perhaps a clear and open revelation of the financial structure of the program from the very first would have dispelled many of these questions.

Problems of recruitment. The major unresolved problem in the Houston program was the recruitment of community participants and retention of community members once recruited. Without the consistent participation of community members, especially those from minority and dissident groups, the maintenance of a meaningful program is not possible. The police were ordered to attend the sessions and had no choice but to attend. While they were paid a token sum ($54 for 18 hours), this fee probably did not adequately compensate those officers who held jobs outside their regular tour of duty. Officers resented the failure of the community to participate on a consistent basis.

At the outset, the program leaders rather naively expected the community to flock eagerly to the sessions. When this did not occur, a massive community involvement program was initiated. The program was publicized via radio, TV, and the local newspapers, the citizens were exhorted to attend the meetings with the time and place being listed. The Houston Council on Human Relations[4] played a central role in recruitment of community participants and in arrangements for scheduling sessions in neighborhood areas. Social clubs, civic clubs, YMCA groups, churches, and the NAACP assisted in recruitment. Unfortunately, although many organizations and individuals representing various segments of the population expressed interest and promised to participate, their cooperation often failed to materialize. Even door to door solicitation often failed to produce participants in a consistent manner.

Community members gave many reasons for their reluctance to participate. Some needed transportation, so buses were made available. Some expressed fear of entering the Police Academy where the meetings were first held, so sessions were scheduled in community centers in the ghetto areas. Some could not make daytime sessions, so classes were scheduled for the evenings. Some claimed never to have heard of the program, so announcements were made in the news media, posted on community bulletin boards, and published in neighborhood newspapers. Despite these arrangements, community participation and attendance remained unsolved problems.

Attendance at the first group meeting with the police is usually good and the interaction heated. Many community members apparently come, however, to express their grievances and blow off steam. Once this has been accomplished, there seems to be little incentive to continue and community attendance dwindles as the weeks pass by. Sometimes it is apparent that community members come only for the purpose of harassing the police in a negative manner and leave when this aim has been accomplished. For example, an organized group of black militants descended on one meeting and engaged the police in a heated recitation of complaints and verbal abuse. However, when the group leader finally called a halt to the flow of invectives and suggested that the group now consider possible constructive solutions to these complaints, the militants abruptly departed from the meeting. These hit and run tactics employed by some community participants were especially difficult to control.

The early phase of any prolonged group interaction is characterized by distrust, while later phases tend to be more open and trusting. Time and

[4]Reverend John P. Murray, formerly Director, Houston Council on Human Relations, was untiring in his efforts to obtain community participation.

continuity of group membership are needed to permit the building of trust and cohesion within a group so that more constructive problem-solving activities can take place. The premature departure of some community members from the present group sessions seriously interfered with the trust building phase of the group process.

A good deal of staff time was consumed in deliberations about how to motivate community attendance, including the possibility of paid attendance for the citizens as well as the police. This solution was abandoned as likely to raise more problems than it solved, not the least of which was obtaining the wherewithal. In the final analysis, it was felt that the only binding inducement to community participation was the meaningful group relationship established by each group leader, so that the citizen could gain a feeling of identification with his group and involvement with his community.

Selection of group leaders. Effective group leaders for this kind of community action program need personal attributes that would tax the resources of an Eagle Scout. The leader must be poised and mature, experienced and skillful in handling difficult groups, intuitive, inventive, and resourceful. He needs the hide of an elephant and "patience sovereign o'er transmuted ill." Previous experience working with poverty groups, minority representatives, and ethnic subgroups is vital. A third of the present group leaders were themselves minority group members, and these leaders appeared to enjoy a decided advantage in working both with the community and police.

Attrition among group leaders in the Houston program was high, with only a very few remaining active in the program throughout its entirety. Leaders gave a number of reasons for resigning, chief among these the emotionally exhausting strain of the sessions and the lack of visible reward, from either police or community, in the form of recognition of the positive contribution made by the program. The repetitious and monotonous character of both the process and content of the sessions was another frequently mentioned detraction. Each six-week session carried a certain deadly encore of issues already dealt with in preceding laboratories. It was difficult for group leaders to build up interest and enthusiasm in still another round of righteous accusations by the community and massive denials by the police.

Some group leaders withdrew from the program because they could not stand the hostility expressed within their group: hostility they assumed to be directed at them personally. These leaders failed to recognize that the hostility, whether expressed by the police or community, was not a personal attack on the leader, but rather for what the leader represented as an agent of change. The group leader threatened the group because he threatened the beliefs and position maintained by each group member. The experienced leader was able to interpret this process for group members and focus their attention on their own resistance to change.

Most people experience some ambivalence toward authority, especially authority as represented by a police officer. Psychologists are no exception and, in fact, because of their own usually liberal social-political values which are often at variance with those held by the police, psychologists may have a particularly difficult time conducting themselves in an unbiased fashion in police-community groups. In the Houston program, the values conflict for some leaders was expressed in their goal of exposing police (but not community) prejudices. Weekly staff meetings in which group leaders' problems were discussed were crucial in helping some leaders recognize and work through their role conflicts. However, the group leader tended to remain the man in the middle in what the police and community viewed as a win or lose situation. The police were inclined to regard the psychologist leader as pro-community and minority group biased, while the participating community often held the psychologist to be a tool of the police and the "Establishment."

Open vs. closed groups. The present program operated with a system of open meetings. That is, community participation was open to all interested citizens and new group members were admitted to any sessions. The police group membership remained constant for all sessions. A system of open meetings carries certain advantages and certain offsetting disadvantages. Open meetings relieve the program administrators of the onerous task of establishing selection criteria or priority lists for community participation. It permits a more democratic atmosphere. When community participation lags, it is a relief to admit anyone to the program who is willing to walk in.

But open meetings interfere with the process of group development, cohesion, and trust, disrupt the continuity of the program, and necessitate the repetition of material and topics already disposed of in prior sessions. Open meetings invite the participation of extremists from both ends of the political spectrum. Political extremists are welcome if they are willing to participate in a meaningful dialogue. However, they usually bring to the meeting a closed mind and a single point of view which they are unwilling to put aside. In the present program, black militants usually arrived only to curse and criticize the police, and left when the group leader attempted to turn the session toward more constructive goals. Extreme right wing white citizens came only to maintain the status quo, "support the local police", and to take copious notes for the purpose of publishing slanted and captious articles about the program.

The problem of open or closed community meetings remains unresolved. Closed meetings offer the best opportunity for the development of group continuity and the orderly pursuit of group problem resolution. If the problem of continued and consistent community participation can be overcome, closed meetings offer the optimum in group structure.

Impact of the New Media

As the Houston program progressed, it attracted the attention of national and international news media. Descriptive articles appeared in such national publications as *Time, Ebony, The National Observer,* and *U. S. News and World Report.* The American Broadcasting Company devoted a one hour TV "Special" to the program, consisting mainly of a video tape of one police-community group meeting. The British Broadcasting Company also taped a police-community group for presentation on the BBC-TV.

All of this publicity had an effect on the program and on the participants, city officials, group leaders, and program sponsors. The spotlight of attention was no doubt flattering to the police and community participants. The focus of national and international attention probably underlined the importance and seriousness of the program and emphasized the fact that the behavior of police and community members was not solely a topic of local concern, but also was open to a far wider audience.

The news media worded its articles in such a way as to create the impression that the primary goal of the program was to identify and root out racial prejudice among the police. Categorizing the program in this way placed a totally unwarranted, one-sided emphasis on its goals.

Over the protests and cautioning of the program administrators, the news media insisted on referring to the police-community meetings as "group psychotherapy." This was particularly upsetting to the police because of the implication that in order to be involved in therapy one must be mentally ill. It placed an uncalled-for burden on the police, who were already on the defensive and sensitive about the group interaction. The news media demonstrated no spirit of responsibility or self-restraint in this respect, since reporters continued to headline their stories in this fashion despite specific requests by the program administrators to desist.

Summary

Has the exposure of nearly 1400 police officers and a corresponding number of community members been worth the time, money, and effort expended? Despite the setbacks and the sometimes contrary results of individual laboratories, the consensus of the participating staff, the city administrators, and the business patrons providing financial support has been cautiously affirmative. Participating community members offer enthusiastic testimonials regarding the effectiveness of the program in promoting, on their part, a more personal and humanistic view of the police officer. No claim is made that 18 hours of discussion and interaction will sweep away years of rancor and distrust. Tension and misunderstanding still exist. But such confrontation and dialogue open the way to greater mutual respect and a more cooperative relationship between police and community.

References

Adams, D. A context for tragedy. *The Texas Observer*, June 9-23, 1967.

Bard, M. & Berkowitz, B. Training police as specialists in family crisis intervention: A community psychology action program. *Community Mental Health Journal*, 1967, **3** (4), 315-17.

Blake, R. R., Mouton, J. S., & Sloma, R. L. The union-management intergroup laboratory: Strategy for resolving intergroup conflict. *The Journal of Applied Behavioral Science*, 1, No. 1, 1965.

Cohen, J. & Struening, E. L. Opinions about mental illness in the personnel of two large mental hospitals. *Journal of Abnormal and Social Psychology*, 1962, **64**, 349-60.

Hanson, P. G., Rothaus, P., Johnson, D. L. & Lyle, F. A. Autonomous groups in human relations training for psychiatric patients. *Journal of Applied Behavioral Science*, 1966, **2**, 305-23.

Helmer, B. Nightmare in Houston. *The Texas Observer*, June 9-23, 1967. *Houston Chronicle*, September 6, 1968.

Justice, B. Detection of potential community violence. Dissemination document, Grant 207 (5.044) Office of Law Enforcement Assistance, U. S. Department of Justice, Washington, D. C., 1968.

Mills, R. B. Innovations in police selection and training. In M. P. Sikes (Chm.), Innovations in police techniques. Symposium presented at the American Psychological Association, San Francisco, 1968.

National Commission on Law Observance and Enforcement. (Wickersham Commission) *Report on lawlessness in law enforcement.* Washington, D. C.: U. S. Government Printing Office, 1931.

President's Commission on Civil Rights. *To secure these rights.* New York: Simon & Schuster, 1947.

Saal, I. Police-community relations: Program models. Unpublished summary of police-community relations programs funded by the Office of Juvenile Delinquency and Youth Development, Social and Rehabilitation Service, U. S. Department of Health, Education and Welfare, December 1967.

Sanford, F. Psychology and the mental health movement. *The American Psychologist*, 1958, **13**, 80-85.

Sikes, M. P. Houston Cooperative Crime Prevention Program. Paper presented at conference on urban minorities and social justice, Southern Methodist University, Dallas, Texas, November 10-11, 1967.

Sikes, M. P. & Cleveland, S. E. Human relations training for police and community. *The American Psychologist*, 1968, **23**, 766-69.

State Advisory Committees. *The Fifty States Report*. Submitted to the Commission on Civil Rights, Washington, D. C.: U. S. Government Printing Office, 1961.

U. S. Riot Commission. (Kerner Commission) *Report of the National Advisory Commission on Civil Disorders*. New York: Bantam Books, 1968.

Chapter 5

Perspectives in Experimental Clinical Psychology

Brendan A. Maher

Most chroniclers of the recent history of clinical psychology in the United States have taken the Boulder Conference (Raimy, 1950) as one of the landmarks by which other developments might be placed in perspective. The conclusions that were reached in that conference have been subject to many subsequent reappraisals, and the debate about the proper training of the clinical psychologist continues almost undiminished. For the purposes of this discussion, it may be of advantage to review briefly the state of affairs in clinical psychology immediately following the Boulder Conference, in order that we might better examine the developments that we see at the present time, of which the contributors to this symposium represent outstanding examples.

By the early 1950's, the field of clinical psychology was characterized by certain features, scientific and professional. Professionally, the principal and vexed question was that of the qualifications necessary to perform individual psychotherapy. Diagnosis and research had been generally conceded by psychiatry to be appropriate functions for the psychologist, but psychotherapy was largely the domain of the psychiatrist. Psychotherapy was more or less synonymous with psychoanalysis. Although alternative approaches had been developed, notably, the client-centered techniques of Carl Rogers and some nascent approaches to conditioning therapy, psychoanalytic or "psychoanalytically oriented" therapies were predominant in most academic departments of psychiatry, and hence in most of the institutions wherein the novice clinical psychologist received his internship training. In spite of the fact that this heavy emphasis upon psychodynamic therapies made nonsense of the view that medical (i.e., biological) training was an important prolegomenon to work in psychotherapy, psychiatry wielded the power of the medical establishment. Not surprisingly, it almost always came out ahead in various interprofessional skirmishes regarding the right to do psychotherapy. The fact that this particular scene has changed, and clinical psychologists now perform psychotherapeutic functions almost everywhere, is more of a tribute to the practical pressures of manpower shortages in the mental health fields than to the enlightenment of psychiatry or the diplomatic skill of psychology.

However, before this evolution had taken place, one of the typical responses of the frustrated clinical psychologist was the establishment of a clinic within an academic setting. In these clinics, no psychiatric hegemony was present and it became possible for the Ph.D. psychologist to follow his psychotherapeutic bent with relative autonomy. Even this situation had its pitfalls. Practical applied psychology lived in an uneasy relationship with other kinds of academic psychology. The research implications of the Doctor of Philosophy degree were a source of friction when clinical curricula were discussed with experimental colleagues. Matters of promotion and tenure for clinical colleagues who were not researching and publishing became foci of acrimony in many graduate departments. The effects of this tension have been discussed often elsewhere and the resolution of the problem is not yet clearly at hand.

Notwithstanding these difficulties, the common-law marriage of clinical and experimental psychology did not always produce offspring which sided with one parent against the other. While many graduate students received their doctorates with a feeling of relief that the research "requirement" was now safely behind them, some were attracted by the exciting possibilities that research training had opened up to them. Sophisticated in the techniques of research design and statistical analysis and familiar with the concepts of general experimental psychology (including physiological psychology), they retained their enthusiasm for the task of applying these concepts and procedures to the problems of psychopathology that had brought them into clinical psychology initially.

Speculations of the kind that begin, "What would have happened if . . . ," are often unprofitable. Still, it is instructive to consider that the current development of experimental psychopathology owes some of its genesis to the inhospitable reception accorded by psychiatry to hopeful psychologist-therapists.

But this is a topic for later discussion and, in the immediate post-Boulder era, the research directions taken by academic clinical psychologists were oriented largely to practical problems of diagnosis and treatment and, to a lesser extent, that of etiology. In the summary that follows here, it is possible only to mention major trends: many interesting lines of research will be omitted from discussion because, although scientifically significant, they were not typical of the general directions that existed at the time.

Without doubt one of the major preoccupations of the researching clinical psychologist in the 1950's was the problem of the validity of psycho-diagnostic instruments. Central to this preoccupation was a concern with the so-called "projective techniques," in particular. Rotter (1963) has noted that the close of World War II marked a shift of interest on the part of the diagnostician, from the measurement of intelligence or other mental abilities, to a concern with motivation — mainly presumed to be unconscious — or with the determination of a psychiatric label for the hospital patient.

The theoretical assumptions that underlay the use of these techniques — mainly, the Rorschach and Thematic Apperception Tests — were often opaque and generally heterogeneous. Hence the kinds of validity that were sought were fundamentally empirical. Did the inferences about oral dependency made from the Rorschach protocol seem to have validity when compared with similar inferences made by other techniques? Questions of this sort were frequently asked with only the sketchiest theoretical articulation of the concepts of "oral dependency" or the like and, as a consequence, considerable lack of clarity about acceptable validity criteria. Often the psychiatric interview was assumed to have a kind of unchallenged validity, and thus to be the touchstone against which the inferences from projective techniques were to be proved. When the task of the diagnostician was to provide a nosological label, the supremacy of psychiatric assessment was readily assumed for validity testing purposes.

Similar efforts went into the investigation of the validity of intelligence test performance profiles in the detection of organic damage, equally handicapped by a purely empirical approach and a serious gap in our basic knowledge of brain-behavior relations. As this effort was of great importance in the development of approaches to the problem of mental retardation, it is of special significance in this volume to note the historical documentation provided in Professor Zigler's contribution, and the direction that has been taken in more recent years.

From the vantage point of the late 1960's, one cannot help but stand slightly aghast at the enormous labor that went into this kind of research and the melancholy results that it produced. The pertinent literature is largely a record of failure and disappointment and has had its own effects upon subsequent developments in clinical psychology. For some investigators, the conclusion to be drawn was inescapable. Available research methodology was too crude to encompass the subtleties of clinical inference; the projective method was obviously valid and the failure must be laid at the door of clumsy and naive investigators.

Others decided that the solution lay, not in better methods, but in a new epistemology whereby the definition of evidence would be changed to remove the inconveniences of current standards of proof. Yet others perceived that better diagnosis would have to wait on better theoretical formulations of etiology, and postponed work on problems of psychopathology returning, instead, to the study of general personality theory.

Oddly enough, all of this had very little influence upon the actual practices of many psychodiagnosticians, who continued to use projective techniques with a blitheness that suggested an unfamiliarity with the literature of their profession. It is hardly an exaggeration to comment that validity investigations did not bring about the demise of projective testing; it has been the decline of projective testing that has brought validity testing into desuetude. As manpower pressures opened up opportunities for clinical psychologists to perform psychotherapy, their interest in diagnostic testing diminished: as this took place, the eternal hunt for validity simply became irrelevant.

The very process that created this irrelevancy was destined, in the long run, to raise the validity issue again more forcefully and in a different form. Entry into the ranks of the psychotherapists was, for psychologists, a prelude to yet another disillusionment: one which they would, however, share with their colleagues, the psychiatrists. In the mid-1950's, there began to appear a trickle of research studies with the disquieting implication that dynamic psychotherapy was — to a large extent — a waste of time. From the provocative figures provided by Eysenck (1952) to the social analysis of the "functional autonomy" of psychotherapy offered by Astin (1961), it was becoming disturbingly clear that the acquisition of the role of psycho-therapist did not necessarily bring with it a justification for an increment in self-esteem. The efficacy of therapeutic treatments now took the place of test-validities as the critical issue in clinical psychology.

Insofar as the evidence accumulated that the traditional psychotherapies were relatively ineffective, the question, once again, became that of the validity of the hypotheses about psychopathology that had inspired the therapy in the first place. Faced with the fact that psychoanalytic therapies were largely useless with hospitalized psychotics, the conclusion was reached that either the patients were "too far gone" to be curable, or that the technique used in treatment was based upon false notions about the etiology of psychosis.

What we might fairly call "the crisis in psychotherapy" was exacerbated by two other developments. One of these, somewhat ironically, was the study by Margaret Rioch and her associates (1963) suggesting that not only was medical training unnecessary as a propaedeutic to training in psychotherapy, but that an intelligent college graduate housewife could acquire the technical procedures of the therapist with relative speed and skill. Nothing was said here about the efficacy of the therapy in which they were trained but, more simply, that they could perform the procedures with an adroitness indistin-guishable from that of more conventionally educated therapists. The fuller implications of this finding have been spelled out in the important book by Schofield (1964), *Psychotherapy: The Purchase of Friendship.*

A second development had been a long time in the making, and may be summarily referred to as the "rise of the behavior therapies." Some ideas are born before their time, and the concepts of the conditioning therapies stood in the wings of the psychotherapeutic stage for some decades, before edging into their contemporary position in the limelight. Pioneers such as Jones (1924), and Watson and Rayner (1920) had already prepared the ground for what was to come later, but it was not until the late 1950's that the work of Wolpe, Eysenck, and the Skinnerians began to enter into prominence.

The history of the period in question is as interesting for what did not happen as for what did. Perhaps the most striking aspect of this period is the nearly total eclipse of biological psychology in the field of clinical psychology. Apart from the acknowledgment that certain neurological disorders required a biological approach in diagnosis, it was widely accepted that the so-called "functional" disorders could safely be understood without reference to biological factors. This state of affairs could be traced to the influence of psychoanalytic theory, on the one hand, and the accumulation of failures in the record of attempts to find biological origins for major psychoses such as schizophrenia. Kallman's work, which stood as a bone in the throat of purely environmental explanations of psychosis, was subject to a deluge of criticism on methodological grounds. Some of it was merited; some of it came strangely from quarters where the application of method-ological criticism to dynamic formulations provoked allegations of "resis-tance" and other nonrational responses. A brazen double standard was applied in evaluating the biological or genetic evidence vs. environmental evidence. In the first case, the hypothesis was assumed to be false until proved true beyond a shadow of a doubt; in the second, the hypothesis was assumed to be true until proved false in all its aspects. Meehl (1962) has analyzed the situation in a now-classic paper.

Untenable positions, like crumbling fortresses, are rarely abandoned until there is a better place to go. Antibiology received its first major setback with the advent of psychopharmacology. Willy-nilly, it was hard to deny that patients treated pharmocologically were often much better, on a day to day basis, than patients undergoing psychotherapy or even than patients who had finished undergoing psychotherapy. Although the rationale for psycho-pharmacological treatment was empirical (in the archaic and pejorative sense), it possessed practical advantages. From a historical point of view, what may turn out to be more important is that it created great difficulties for those who would try to continue to deny the role of biological factors in psychological mood states and their behavioral elements. The attempt was made and some psychodynamicists made gallant efforts to interpret the tranquilizers in terms of their unconscious significance rather than their molecular structure. Gallant or not, they were fighting a losing battle. Biology was back to stay.

While the influence of drug therapies was evident at once — socially, almost instantaneously — other developments in biology were occurring, the effects of which were not at first apparent. Perhaps the most profound of these was the discovery of the functions of the reticular activating system. Many scientists shared in this work but, for archival purposes, we may regard the report of Moruzzi and Magoun (1949) as one of the early landmarks. By opening up new vistas of the relationship between biology and states of consciousness, it became possible to revive the discussion of the mind-body problem with additional insights; it also raised the possibility that disturbed states of consciousness might have a biological basis, hitherto unsuspected outside the known phenomena of the toxic psychoses and neurological diseases of the senium.

Although the specific events in biological psychology were circumscribed — drugs and reticular physiology — their development created an atmosphere in which psychobiological thinking became respectable once more, and not merely an atavism to be found only in anachronistic European departments of psychiatry! In this atmosphere, it became possible to look at the biology of schizophrenia with renewed interest (and less naivete) and to turn the same kind of attention to the character disorders, the depressions, and other "functional" syndromes. Some of the results of this can be seen in Hare's report in this volume.

While the successes of pharmacology might have pulled some psycho-pathologists in a biotropic direction, the failures of individual psychotherapy had pushed others in sociotropic fashion. As the treatment of individual psychotics by psychodynamic methods seemed to be relatively unprofitable, the logic of psychodynamic theories of etiology has led some psycho-therapists to concentrate upon the continuing parent-child interactions of the patient and his family, in the hope that the rectification of these might lead to alleviation of the sufferings of the patient. Hence the development of emphasis upon the concepts of schizophrenogenesis, assigned to one or both parents as a quasi-abusive adjective, and the inevitable growth of the techniques of family therapy. Not all of the work in this area has stemmed from psychodynamic propositions: behaviorally oriented therapists have long been interested in techniques whereby the parent is educated in the principles of reinforcement and extinction (e.g., Rotter, 1954) and in understanding the relationship between behavior and the consequences that follow it.

It will be apparent that the lines dividing recent history from present activity and present activity from the near future are, at best, tenuous. However, for present purposes it will be useful to draw a line at this point and venture some estimates of the future.

Behavior Change Techniques

No crystal ball is needed to foresee the continued rapid rate of expansion of the conditioning therapies. The year 1969 witnessed the publication of two major textbooks on the topic (Yates, 1969; Franks, 1969), the foundation of a new journal in the United States (an event preceded by a similar development in Great Britain, some years before), as well as a continued increase in the rate at which other contributions appear in the scientific and professional literature. Reflecting this interest has been the establishment of a special interest section of the American Psychological Association (Section III of Division 12) with a membership of nearly 200 at the time of writing.

The growth of interest and scientific contribution has been hampered, however, by a dearth of training facilities. At the end of 1969, formal training was available at only a handful of institutions.[1] Much training continues to be of an *ad hoc* kind or to depend on self-training. The pressure of demand for such training will undoubtedly lead to an increase in suitable facilities, as and when public funds make this expansion possible.

A significant aspect of this expansion is likely to include the training of members of other professions, neighborhood workers, parents, etc., in the use of behavioral principles in their work. Notable beginnings have already been made in this respect. Bearing in mind that the solution to the problem of behavior disorders demands a massive application of manpower beyond the capacity of the mental health professions to provide, it appears inevitable that we should expect an emphasis upon techniques that require relatively brief periods of treatment, are effective, are readily transferable to the social habitat of the patient, and involve skills that can be acquired by intelligent people in and out of the professional circles that ordinarily deal with the patient. In fact, the kinds of considerations that created a favorable reception for nondirective techniques apply with equal force to the reception of behavioral therapy, but with the added advantage that the question of therapeutic effectiveness has been answered with more reassurance.[2]

Caveats have been uttered by several sources against the dangers of orthodoxy and establishmentarianism in the conditioning therapies. These dangers are not entirely chimerical: we have had ample opportunity to witness their sterilizing effect upon the fruitfulness of Freudian psychology. The remedy is available in the continuance of the emphasis upon the role of experimental research (rather than clinical observation) in providing correctives for undue optimism or parochial insistence upon specific theoretical propositions. A firm locus within the framework of experimental psychology is the most reliable protection against the development of authoritarianism in theory and practice.

Turning to biological therapies, it seems clear that the next few years will include an increase in the attempt to provide a sounder psychobiological basis for the present empirical use of drugs. Such advances are inevitably dependent upon advances in neuropsychology, generally, and upon new

---

[1] The University of Illinois, The University of Wisconsin, Stanford University, The State University of New York at Stony Brook, and Temple University Medical School.

[2] In this connection, we should also expect that behavioral-therapeutic procedures that are self-administerable, employing automated devices, teaching-machine techniques etc., should appear in increasing numbers.

knowledge in the biology of psychopathology, specifically. There are signs that the problems of biology and behavior will receive attention from biological scientists to a greater extent than has been the case hitherto. The impetus for this comes, in part, from the fact that molecular biology and structural genetics have made enormous strides in the last decade, coupled with the increased sophistication with which problems of behavioral genetics and epidemiology have been tackled during the same period.

It is more difficult to be sanguine about the long-term implications of the activities that are currently subsumed under the heading "community psychology". Mention has already been made of the revised view of therapeutic strategy that leads to consultation and intervention in the school, the family, and the social habitat of the client, generally. While terms such as "intervention" and "consultation" have an attractive tone to them, the fact remains that the consultant or intervener must be possessed of a technology that makes his efforts more successful than the application of common sense alone might be. Or, put another way, the results of a community procedure can be no better than the validity of the principles upon which the procedure is based. Advice directed to teachers, for example, that is derived from psychodynamic notions of child development will be no better and no worse than the validity of these notions themselves. The fact that the therapist is labeled a "consultant" and works directly with the school authorities rather than exclusively with the child or parents does not necessarily lead us to expect any greater efficacy than that which has been reported from traditional clinical models of treatment. At the present time, there has been much discussion in the literature about the manner in which consultation might be arranged and consultants be trained (e.g., Kelly, 1964), but very little serious discussion about the theoretical orientation and practical techniques that might be used. It is possible to wonder whether or not the concept of community mental health depends upon a false analogy to medical public health. Public health, as exemplified by such practices as mass inoculation, quarantine, preventative diet programs, and well-baby clinics, is based upon solid scientific knowledge relating to the prevention of disease. At the present time, there is grave doubt as to whether or not psychopathology has progressed to the point at which we can make confident statements about the prevention of neurotic or psychotic breakdown. Until this information is available, the community mental health approach may be confined to bringing conventional therapeutic principles to bear in dealing with existing disorders, but at an earlier stage in their development than is usually found in the clinic. And here, as mentioned already, the results can be no better than the validity of the therapies that are being applied.

All in all, it seems probable that the application of *experimental* principles to the study of community mental health practices will be difficult to achieve, in any event. Problems of control populations, differing diagnostic standards, the tendency of preventative programs to become case-finding programs, and a host of other variables make it peculiarly difficult to evaluate the success of preventative measures in any meaningful way, except over very long periods of time. A decade ago, the World Health Organization (W.H.O., 1960) remarked on the need for the use of controlled studies in general problems of the epidemiology of mental illness, but the succeeding years have produced few instances of the application of experimental control to investigations of incidence, prevalence, or preventative efficacy.

Etiology

Therapeutic techniques do not depend, of necessity, upon a valid knowledge of etiology. Preventative measures do to a much greater extent. Although the use of conditioning techniques may be expected to increase as a therapeutic strategy, the study of etiology may be expected to develop in several different directions. One of the major possibilities is the study of individual differences in susceptibility to the acquisition of various kinds of learning. Differences of this kind might be explicable in terms of biological endowments, a kind of explanation that revives interest in the concept of temperament; alternatively, some of these differences might well be a function of early learning. If we accept the proposition that individual differences in the acquisition of anxiety are key factors in the explanation of neurotic development, then the biological processes of central interest are those governing visceral response patterns. Elsewhere in this volume, Hare has touched upon the role of these responses in the character disorders, and other works report the importance of these in depression (e.g., Mendels, 1970) and schizophrenia (e.g., Venables, 1964).

Investigations of visceral functioning have been limited, until recently, by laboratory restrictions upon the operation of the polygraph. Newer developments in radio-telemetry have made it possible to study visceral patterns in the natural habitat (e.g., Maher, 1966) and we may expect that the use of this technique will increase as certain matters of engineering and cost are resolved. In any event, we may expect to see the steady growth of information pertinent to the role of temperament in the acquisition of neurosis and the determination of its symptomatology. This position has been anticipated for several years by the theoretical and experimental work of Eysenck (1947, 1962). Although the specific dimensions of temperament that he has adduced may not command agreement as to their central significance in the understanding of neurosis, Eysenck's emphasis upon temperamental variables in psychopathology (first mentioned systematically by Pavlov) will undoubtedly be shared by experimental clinicians in the decades ahead.

Turning to the psychoses, it seems to be increasingly clear that the major emphases in investigation will be placed upon the psychobiology of consciousness and related disorders of attention and cognition. Applications of this view to schizophrenia are already well-begun (e.g., Fish, 1961; Venables, 1964) and many phenomena that have been recalcitrant to systematic explanation are now amenable to investigation in these terms. A casual reading of the history of attempts to locate a biological pathogen for schizophrenia might well induce pessimism about the prospects for further work along these lines. Kety (1959) reported a review of biological and genetic investigations of schizophrenia, in terms that have been widely misinterpreted as justifying a reflection of biological theories altogether. It is useful here to quote directly from his paper.

> Although *the evidence for genetic and therefore biological factors as important and necessary components in the etiology of many or all of the schizophrenias is quite compelling,* the sign posts pointing the way to their discovery are at present quite blurred. . . . (p.1595. Italics added)

Blurred though the sign posts may be, the evidence is, as Kety points out, compelling, and it is the compelling nature of the evidence that leads us to assume that the interrelations between psychology and biology in this matter will grow closer.

Etiology implies diagnosis. The desuetude into which traditional diagnostic testing has already fallen is likely to continue. From the behavior therapist's point of view, the task of diagnosis is encompassed by the procedures of behavioral analysis. The differences between the methods of behavioral analysis and those of conventional testing for psychodynamic constellations have been well summarized by Kanfer and Saslow (1965). They point out that this approach is not a substitute for assignment of the patient to categories, which may be desirable for statistical, administrative, or research purposes, but "is intended to replace other diagnostic formulations purporting to serve as a basis for making decisions about specific therapeutic interventions." As behavior therapies continue to expand, the justification for dynamic patterns of explanation declines, and with it much of the rationale for testing aimed at providing inferences about psychodynamics.

Psychobiological explanations of psychopathology tend to turn the diagnostician towards laboratory measures of basic psychological processes. Measures of attention, motivation, learning deviations, information-processing deficits, and the like, come to have the relationship to psychopathology that the analysis of blood, measures of intestinal function, and other laboratory techniques have to physical pathology. It is quite possible that some day biological measures alone will have diagnostic value, but that day seems rather remote at present.

Professional Education

It has been the purpose of this chapter to examine some recent developments in experimental clinical psychology and to speculate about the future direction in which they may lead us. In staying within this rubric, it has been possible, so far, to ignore the fact that many clinical psychologists are unsympathetic to the experimental point of view when it is applied to the problems that interest them. Consequently, the very developments that point to an increasing importance for the role of experimental thinking in clinical psychology, also presage a widening rift between this view of things and the view held by more traditional clinicians. By traditional here is meant the model that emphasizes the technique of face-to-face psychotherapy, psychodynamic explanations, and the use of clinical observation as a basis for validating hypotheses.

It should be noted that the kind of difference referred to here is not one between academic-research psychologists and applied-practicing psychologists. It is between experimental-behavioristic-biopsychology, on the one hand, in both its research and clinical applications, vs. clinical-psychodynamic-antibiological psychology, on the other. This latter formulation is already a little out of date and should be expanded to include the recent movements towards new varieties of group psychotherapy (nude therapy, some kinds of sensitivity training, marriage fighting, and other exotic flora on the nether borders of professional irrationality). However veridical this dichotomy may be, there is no doubt that the chronic issue of clinical training, referred to in the opening lines of this chapter, is as subject as ever to acrimonious debate. It would be impossible to speculate in any comprehensive way now on the directions that training in clinical psychology will take. What may be suggested is that, in some centers at least, there will develop programs designed to equip the clinical psychologist to take advantage of and contribute to the kinds of progress in biopsychology that have been suggested herein.

We may, therefore, look for programs in which exposure to the principles and practice of behavior therapy, knowledge of psychopharmacology, behavior genetics, personality research, experimental psychopathology, neuropsychology, and epidemiology will come to the fore, while diagnostic testing, individual psychotherapy, and the study of global personality theory will be of minor importance. These new programs may well find themselves at odds with other programs in clinical psychology, but more at ease with the life sciences generally, and experimental psychology in particular.

REFERENCES

Astin, A. W. The functional autonomy of psychotherapy. *American Psychologist*, 1961, 16, 75-78.

Eysenck, H. J. *Dimensions of personality.* London: Routledge & Kegan Paul, 1947.

Eysenck, H. J. The effects of psychotherapy: An evaluation. *Journal of Consulting Psychology*, 1952, 16, 319-24.

Eysenck, H. J. Conditioning and personality. *British Journal of Psychology*, 1962, 53, 299-305.

Fish, F. A. A neurophysiological theory of schizophrenia. *Journal of Mental Science*, 1961, 107, 828-38.

Franks, C. M. *Behavior therapy: Appraisal and status.* New York: McGraw-Hill, 1969.

Jones, M. C. The elimination of children's fears. *Journal of Experimental Psychology*, 1924, 7, 382-90.

Kanfer, F. H. & Saslow, G. Behavioral analysis: An alternative to diagnostic classification. *Archives of General Psychiatry*, 1965, 12, 529-38.

Kelley, J. G. The mental health agent in the urban community. *Urban America in the planning of mental health services.* New York: Group for Advancement in Psychiatry, 1964. Pp. 474-94.

Kety, S. S. Biochemical theories of schizophrenia. Part II. *Science*, 1959, 129, 1590-96.

Maher, B. A. *Principles of psychopathology: An experimental approach.* New York: McGraw-Hill, 1966.

Meehl, P. E. Schizotaxia, schizotypy, schizophrenia. *American Psychologist*, 1962, 17, 827-38.

Mendels, J. *Affective disorders.* New York: Wiley, 1970

Moruzzi, G. & Magoun, H. W. Brainstem reticular formation and activation of the EEG. *EEG and Clinical Neurophysiology*, 1949, 1, 455-73.

Raimy, V. C. (Ed.). *Training in clinical psychology.* (Boulder Conference) Englewood Cliffs, N. J.: Prentice-Hall, 1950.

Rioch, M. J., Elkes, C., Flint, A. A., Udansky, B. S., Newman, R. G., & Silber, E. National Institute of Mental Health pilot study in training mental health counselors. *American Journal of Orthopsychiatry*, 1963, 33, 678-89.

Rotter, J. B. *Social learning and clinical psychology.* Englewood Cliffs, N. J.: Prentice-Hall, 1954.

Rotter, J. B. A historical and theoretical analysis of some broad trends in clinical psychology. In S. Koch (Ed.), *Psychology: A study of a science.* New York: McGraw-Hill, 1963.

Schofield, W. *Psychotherapy: The purchase of friendship.* Englewood Cliffs, N. J.: Prentice-Hall, 1964.

Venables, P. H. Input dysfunction in schizophrenia. In B. A. Maher (Ed.), *Progress in experimental personality research.* Vol. I. New York: Academic Press, 1964.

Watson, J. B. & Rayner, R. Conditioned emotional reactions. *Journal of Experimental Psychology*, 1920, 3, 1-14.

World Health Organization. *Epidemiology of Mental Disorders.* Technical Report No. 185. Geneva W.H.O., 1960.

Yates, A. J. *Behavior therapy.* New York: Wiley, 1969.

Name Index

Achenbach, T. 47, 94, 110
Adams, D. 167, 199
Albert, R.S. 5, 39
Alexander, F. 39
Arieti, S. 36, 39
Aristotle 130
Aronfreed, J. 102, 115
Arthur, R. J. 8, 42
Astin, A. W. 204, 212
Atkinson, J. W. 83, 110
Ax, A. F. 37, 39

Badt, M. I. 97, 110
Baer, D. M. 102, 113
Balla, D. 47, 62, 68, 70, 71, 72,
    75, 103, 104, 105, 110, 120
Bard, M. 167, 199
Barrett, H. E. 101, 110
Bastian, J. 137, 161
Bay-Rakal, S. 8, 39
Beck, S. 156, 161
Bell, R. L. 165
Benson, F. 107, 118
Berkowitz, B. 167, 199
Berkowitz, H. 76, 110
Bernard, J. I. 26, 39
Blake, R. R. 173, 176, 199
Blaylock, J.J. 26, 39
Brigante, T. R. 5, 39
Brown, J. S. 29, 39
Bruner, J. S. 48, 93, 110
Bryan, J. H. 26, 39
Burks, B. S. 106, 110
Burlingham, D. 77, 112
Butterfield, E. C. 66, 68, 75, 76, 84,
    92, 98, 99, 101, 103, 104, 105,
    110, 111, 115, 117, 120
Byck, M. 80, 111

Cameron, A. 78, 79, 111
Capobianco, F. 101, 120
Carlson, F. 1, 40

Carr-Saunders, A. 100, 101, 114
Chapman, J. P. 161
Chapman, L. J. 123, 128, 161
Chase, M. 5, 39
Child, I. 81, 120
Clark, L. P. 62, 111
Clarke, A. D. B. 100, 102, 103, 111
Clarke, A. M. 100, 102, 103, 111
Cleckley, H. 2, 3, 5, 20, 21, 27,
    31, 37, 39
Cleland, C. 97, 111
Cleveland, S. E. 165, 180, 200
Cohen, J. 183, 199
Collman, R. D. 108, 111
Cox, F. 77, 111
Craddick, R. A. 25, 39
Craft, M. J. 1, 39
Craig, K. 38, 39
Cromwell, R. L. 75, 82, 83, 111
Cruse, D. 96, 111
Currie, J. S. 23, 40

Dahlin, Y. 12, 15, 45
Dain, N. 1, 40
Davids, A. 155, 161
Davidson, K. S. 83, 117
Davies, S. P. 53, 94, 107, 109, 112
Davis, A. 78, 80, 112
deLabry, J. 79, 88, 121
Denny, M. R. 97, 112
Dickens, C. 130
Diggory, J. C. 89, 95, 112, 116
Douglas, R. J. 9, 40
Douvan, E. 78, 80, 112
Durkin, K. 79, 118

Edgerton, R. B. 95, 112
Eisenman, R. 26, 39
Elkes, C. 204, 212
Ericson, M. 79, 80, 112
Eron, L. D. 125, 161, 163
Eysenck, H. J. 21, 40, 204, 209, 212

215